Well-Being Ultimatum:

A Self-Care Guide for Strategic Healers -
Those who live in the service, leadership
and healing of others

By Dr. Suzie Carmack,
PhD, MFA, MEd, ERYT, PMA-CPT

DEDICATION

Thank you to my teachers, colleagues, clients and students, especially:

Dr. Gary Kreps, PhD, Dr. Joshua Rosenberger, PhD,
Dr. Don Boileau, PhD, Dr. Anne Nicotera, PhD,
Neva Ingalls, ERYT 500, Lisa Johnson, ERYT 500,
Pamela Sills, Lance Schmeidler, Bill Lynch,
Ava Kennedy, Karen Kraybill, and my
colleagues and students at George Mason University and
The American University

My love to my amazing family, especially

My Dad, Patrick Carmack, who taught me to love and teach
without conditions or judgment

My Sister Cyndi Carmack, who taught me about healing

My Brother Eddie Carmack, who taught me about serving

My Cousin Brenda Wolfram Murn, who taught me to never give up

My Children: Chris, Brandon and Sophia,
who deepened my understanding of what love and joy really mean

The LOML: Bob Shircliff who inspires my subjective and objective well-being,
every single day; thank you for making life really fun

And My Angels
Mother Dixie Lea Reese and Sister Patricia Carmack,
who taught me to savor every day in this lifetime.

CONTENTS

PROLOGUE
My Very Personal Well-being Ultimatum Aha Moment

It's May 2011.

I'm laying on a lumpy platform in a doctor's office, which is trying to pass itself off for a daybed. And this platform would've gotten away with it too, if it had not been for the sheet of paper that is meant to somehow keep the space between myself and the bed allegedly sterile.

I've been on one of these before, but this time I'm not staring at the ceiling.

My head is turned to the right. I can see a female nurse in the corner out of the side of my eyes, when I choose to open them. Right now they're pretty tightly squinted shut. When I see her she is trying to both be there and not be there in the corner. She's not even trying to look busy.

But that's not why I'm squinting so hard.

To my left, a doctor is poking me with a needle in the neck. And then another.

You might think that this is what's bothering me...this giant needle. The rush of chemicals that is sliding down inside my neck. But actually, its something altogether different.

It's bothering me, a lot, that it's quiet.

He's not talking at all, except for a barely audible sigh. I can feel his annoyance with the situation in front of him. I'm trying to be empathetic to his plight, but I'm having a hard time because right now the situation he is annoyed with is Me.

And I'd kinda like to see my kids grow up.

All I can do though is wait for the numbness to kick in while he pinches, prods, and pinches again. I stop feeling the chemicals oozing inside my skin, and it's getting a little foggy in my head.

And then, there it is.

I know he is cutting my skin because I can see the shadow of his arm against the opposite wall.

He's still not talking.

The nurse is not talking.

And I really can't talk...because someone I just met is slicing my neck open.

And I really really want to see my kids grow up. So I better be quiet.

So I'm left to wonder a few things.

Will he cut my carotid artery and save me the worry of wondering if it really is cancer this time? I want to smile at the hypocricy of this thought, but my lower face and jaw are numb now and I might smile too big.

That's funny too actually. Smiling too big because it might be cancer again.

But I can't start laughing, so all I can do is think. I really don't want to go through the "I wish I had lived differently" thoughts. I've done those many times and they really aren't fun.

So I go with the "well, if I do get out of this...I'm going to..." thoughts.

Will I have another scar like the one on my left breast? It will be harder to hide this one I think. That one fits in nicely right under my bathing suit as long as it's not too low cut.

Will I have enough time to finish the paper I have due for tomorrow? Right now I can't remember if it's the response paper on mother-daughter dialogues about breast cancer or the literature review on health literacy. Or maybe I was supposed to grade my undergrads' papers. Right now I can't remember. And it would be difficult to get to the daytimer in my purse that has become my second brain.

What will I feed the kids for dinner tonight? Ordering in seems to be a good idea because if I do survive this I really won't give a shit about whether or not I fit into my jeans this weekend. So Chinese food sounds lovely.

That makes me want to laugh a little. But the thought occurs that he's still cutting and that laughing would not be very funny. Or maybe he's stitching now. It's hard to tell.

All I know is he's still not talking.

If I could talk, I'd tell him that I'm a health communication scholar, yoga teacher, community health strategist and single mother of three. I'd tell him that between these four roles I know enough to know that he should be saying something, ANYTHING to help me make sense of this moment in my life, where I know I may not get to see another day. He could at least be giving me a play-by-play like they do at basketball games.

But I can't finish that thought, because now he's walking around the table and I can see him facing me. He's trying not to make eye contact with me and then he says he's done. And that it was tough. Something about it being a tough area with not a lot of skin. Hard to get the margins. They'll run the sample through the labs. I should come back in a week to find out the results. He walks out. The nurse follows him looking at her chart.

So I guess I have lived through this, I think.

The room is still quiet.

I slowly get up and try to put on my shirt. There's no one in the lobby waiting for me so I head to my car.

And it's hard. And I'm scared. And I'm tired. And I'm worried.

And someone looks at me in the elevator like I'm a little crazy.

And the fogginess is still there, but I know I can snap out of it.

As the doors close and the elevator starts its decent I realize that's what single moms like me do. They snap out of it and they get home in time to make sure there is some type of food for dinner.

And that was it.

Somewhere in that elevator, I had my moment. The moment. The Moment.

A moment where I saw my life from the bottom up. I saw the layers of my worries, my doubts, my joys and my triumphs. I saw the people in my life and what they really, really mean to me and the cold truth of what I really, really, meant to them. And I saw that most of it, well, all of it, really doesn't matter. Not because I thought that it was all a waste – nothing could be further from the truth. I just realized that it's all part of one giant story that I am living in. It's just this part that I'm playing, that is this lifetime.

And I smiled. Because after so many years of studying health and well-being, and teaching others about it, I finally knew. In my heart and in my body and in my mind and in my spirit. It was time to make a well-being ultimatum. With my Self.

This book is for you if you are ready for your moment.

The moment where you start living like you mean it - no excuses - and honoring the truth of who you really are. The moment when you stop making excuses that everyone and everything else comes first -- no matter how big your life is and no matter how many troubles you have. The moment when you start realizing that how you live every day matters for how long you get to stick around here on planet earth, and the quality with which you experience each of those days. The moment when you start taking care of your body – not as a punishment through denial and deprivation but as a respectful act of love and gratitude. Because this is the moment when you start performing joy every day -- in your mind, your body and your life. This is the moment you make your well-being ultimatum.

Oh my heart.
Don't become discouraged so easily.
Have faith.
In the hidden world, there are many mysteries, many wonders.
Even if the whole planet threatens your life, don't let go of the
Beloved's robe for even a breath
— Rumi

If we could change ourselves,
the tendencies in the world would also change.
As a man changes his own nature,
so does the attitude of the world change towards him....

We need not wait to see what others do.
— Gandhi

CHAPTER 1:
SUPER HERO SYNDROME: WHY YOUR DRIVE TO HEAL, LEAD AND/OR SERVE OTHERS CALLS FOR A WELL-BEING ULTIMATUM

Have you ever seen Wonder Woman or Super Man eat, sleep, work out, or go out to dinner with family and friends? They don't need to – or at least they don't think that they do.

News flash: Despite your heroic tendencies – your compelling need to live in the service, leadership and healing of others like Wonder Woman or Super Man – you are human too. Unlike those and many other Super Heroes, you are allowed to ask for help and support so that you can save and change the world. This means that you must put your self-care first -- not after everything else is taken care of, but beforehand. Every day.

Sound familiar? The idea of this is easy for anyone to understand. It's the implementation into our life experience that is the hard part.

Why is that? Why is it that the people who dedicate their life's work to helping (healing) other people have a really hard time beginning with themselves? Why is it that all of us humans need to be reminded on airplanes to put the oxygen mask on ourselves before we take care of the person in need next to us?

If you are curious about these questions, and what they may mean for your life's work, your health and your well-being, then this book is for you.

Let's begin by discussing something called Hero Syndrome. It is a condition which has not been scientifically researched much, but has been discussed at length in popular culture.

> "The hero is driven by the need for approval, recognition, and being wanted and valued. The need is met briefly by the "high" of being asked to do something, but it is exactly this short-lived high that makes it an addictive cycle. In order to get it met, you have to keep saying yes. The secret is getting the need met in a much healthier way. (Fortgang, 1999)

Although there has been a scientific screening instrument (survey) developed to identify those with the Hero Syndrome, there have been no scientific studies conducted to investigate it or to validate the survey which screens for it in the first place. Further research is therefore needed to explore whether or not it is really a syndrome or not, and if so, the syndrome's causes, as well as the ramifications for those who have it.

Despite the fact that the hero syndrome has not been scientifically investigated as well as it should be, I start our discussion on the assumption that it does indeed exist. This is because I have seen the pattern of thinking noted above many times – in my work with clients, students, and even, yes, with myself.

Upon further review of the description of Hero Syndrome, we can see that Hero Syndrome does not sound like something that is very fun. It sounds like something that feels like being overwhelmed by one's need to feel needed – often times without reward.

At first glance we might assume this is just a self-esteem issue – and of course it is. The person is trying so hard to please others they have forgotten to take care of themselves. They may not even know what that means.

This book does not unpack why that might be – why some people have self-esteem issues that highly increase the likelihood that they become "yes people" (heroes). Instead, I propose here, that there is actually a "special case" version of Hero Syndrome, which I call Super Hero Syndrome.

Unlike the hero in Hero Syndrome, who is caught in an endless cycle of people pleasing that never seems to feel right or powerful, the Super Hero has essentially the opposite problem.

In the Super Hero syndrome, the individual not only gets a "high" off of helping other people, they get a second (super) "high" from helping, healing, leading and/or caregiving others. This second high results from the fact that these special case heroes – these Super Heroes – perceive their service-, leadership-, and/or healing-oriented work to be a fundamental component of who they are. Like everyday heroes, they are addicted to saying yes. But unlike everyday heroes, this addiction does not stem from their need for approval; it stems from the fact that they are in positions in which they really are needed (to heal, to lead, to serve, to protect, to counsel, to coach, to give care, and/or to parent).

Simply put -- it's not about their self-esteem, its about their call to service. Super Heroes are tirelessly dedicated to helping others, and they know this work is their life calling and/or their Life's Calling.

To explain further, I propose here that Super Hero syndrome is a "super-charged" version of hero syndrome that can easily plague those working in service-, caregiving-, medical-, military-, leader- and/or healing-related avocations. The folks who are the ones who lead us, who heal us, who protect us, who care for us, and who serve us are more likely to "give and give until they can't" because they have a super-strong sense of "meaning and purpose" regarding what they do. Their desire to help is embedded in who they are. The result is that they can have a super-charged addiction to helping others, because they essentially receive "two hits" every time that they say yes: the high of feeling needed (described in the hero syndrome definition above), plus, the second high of fulfilling their "call" to help the world. As we will see in chapter three, both social support (feeling needed) and meaning and purpose (calling) are types of subjective well-being – they make us feel good (happy) about ourselves, and our lives.

I should note here that Super Hero syndrome, is not only a special case of Hero syndrome, it also has some similarities with

Chronic Hero syndrome. In Chronic Hero syndrome, a clinically-recognized phenomenon, affected people create a risky and/or desperate situation, and/or disobey rules so that they can resolve the situation and be seen as extraordinary.

The difference between Super Heroes and Chronic Heroes, is that Super Heroes do not have any malicious intent in what they do; they do not desire to break civil or ethical laws. However, they may at times create "risky" situations regarding their own health and well-being by ignoring their own real and human needs in favor of their call to serve and heal. And, they may at times believe they are "above the rules" of self-care (i.e. forgoing meals, sleep, exercise) because they perceive that they don't need these as much as "everyday" humans do. They believe that their attention must instead be devoted to their humanitarian work, rather than their self-care. In short, the Super Hero will answer the Call no matter what.

How do you know if you have Super Hero syndrome? Nothing gives you more joy than helping (i.e. serving, leading, teaching, parenting, caregiving or healing) others. Even though the heroic work you do helping others is challenging, and at times exhausting, you love every minute of it. This is because the selfless work that you do helps and/or heals people, and that act of service is your calling. Like a Super Hero, you take this calling seriously; it is not a 9-5 job but it is a 24/7 way of life. You are there when people need you – no matter what. You save the world wherever and however you can, through big choices and small acts.

You, Super Hero, are all about saving the world, one healing (leading, serving, caregiving, parenting) act at a time.

Whether your work is volunteer or paid; and whether it is inside of the home or outside of the home, you want nothing more than to "be the change you wish to see in the world". As a parent, a scholar, a warrior, a CEO, a teacher, a military service member, a police officer, and even a factory worker or a rock star -- you are a change catalyst in your community. Others look to you for guidance, leadership and healing (whether you ask them to or not). And you oblige them because nothing gives you greater joy—seeing *them* happy, safe, and thriving.

If you are a leader, you put your people's needs first. If you are an artist, you see your work as a driver for social change. If you are a caregiver, you are committed to providing that care without question – anytime, day or night. If you are a teacher, you are concerned with your student's ability to learn as much about themselves as your lesson plan. If you are a parent, the kids come first no matter how old they are. If you are a writer, you struggle with syntax until that difficult concept is boiled down to simplicity, perhaps without realizing a few hours have gone by in the process. If you are a clinician, you pull a 24-hour shift because the latest trauma would not wait. You do these things without fail, no matter what it takes out of you, or from you, because that is who you are.

If you want to, and can do any and/or all of these tasks without fail, every day, then you are a healer. I don't wish to imply that there is anything wrong with this type of excellence and/or high performance in these roles.

If, however, you put these tasks first – before your own self-care practices, before your own needs for social support from family and friends, and/or before your need for services that help you to maintain your health, wellness and well-being (physician, dentist, therapist and/or any other type of specialists), then you are suffering from Super Hero syndrome.

The distinction between a healer and a Super Hero, is that the healer is dedicated to helping others in these selfless ways, but does this without sacrificing their own needs in the process. The Super Hero, on the other hand, is so consumed by helping others that they do not always follow through on their self-care, social support and/or service needs. They believe that others need them too much for them to take the time that they need to take care of themselves. They are the one that the flight attendant would be concerned about in a crisis, because they would be the least likely to put their own oxygen mask on before helping the person next to them.

Here's the problem.

When your need to help and heal others gets in the way of your self-care – before the needs you have as a human to sleep; to exercise; to balance your financial priorities; to eat well; to spend quality time with family and friends; to engage the creative aspects of your psyche; and to manage your (medical) health needs effectively – a breakdown in your mind, your body and your life can occur that does not look much different than the effect that kryptonite has on Super Man. In the process of healing, leading and/or serving others without honoring these needs for self-care, you create a risky and potentially threatening situation for your longevity and your quality of life.

How do I know? I know, because for years, I had Super Hero syndrome too, although I didn't have a name for it then and I don't think I would have admitted to it if I had known about it. I thought it was just this "thing" about myself that I could not deny – that putting others first and ignoring my own self-care needs in the process was how I did life, because after all, I was dedicated to my call to service. This "whatever it takes" attitude was reinforced during my formative years in education and throughout my career; people who push hard to get the job done are celebrated for their unwavering commitment to the project at hand.

Successful people are known for getting things done – no matter what it takes.

I was this person. I was the person that got things done. No matter what. If you have seen the jacket to this book, you see I have earned a lot of letters – not because I wanted to collect letters but because each educational venture was something that had value for the (healing) work I was doing at the time, and because I like completing things. I like knowing all I can about something. I am insanely curious, and I don't like quitting. Anything.

This drive I have (and still had) is not all bad. It has enabled me to succeed and to have a mostly wonderful life so far – a life I never would have dreamed of having as a little girl growing up in a suburb of Pittsburgh, PA.

However, the drive had a scary side too. Usually the "get it done no matter what" part of me would be all too willing to ignore my self-care, social support and/or services needs. It wasn't because I didn't value these – I did. This trade of my call to service for my personal (care) needs was made in order to Make. Things. Happen.

The problem (which I did not view as such) persisted because I received nothing but positive support for this behavior. A dangerous cocktail of thinking occurred that went something like this. (1) I felt good helping others, knowing that my work was making a difference for them; (2) I felt as if I was fulfilling my sense of meaning and purpose (service) in the world because I was engaging in healing acts and (3) I received nothing but positive messages of appreciation for my efforts.

What was not to like? I was helping people feel good, and that felt good for me. I was succeeding as far as my work and the world was concerned. But just like any cocktail, what felt good at the time was not completely good for me.

The problem with this line of thinking, was not that I was enjoying the "triple shot" of feel-good feelings from my service-above-self attitude. The problem was found in the fact that I had a strong belief that my self-care could wait (until whatever the task I was working on was completed) and that I didn't need other people's support (even though I was actively supporting them). After all, I was the one people came to when they needed help. I was the one that was calm during insanity and/or crisis events. I was strong, and I was functioning well, and I was helping people -- so why not wait another day to take care of myself when there was so much (healing, leading, serving) work to do? In the case of the teams that I led and/or managed, I did not want them to see me ask for help because this would mean that perhaps I didn't know what I was completely doing after all – and that might make them uncomfortable (which of course made me really uncomfortable).

Not only could my self-care and my need for social support wait, I was also very reluctant to lean on any type of (professional) service that would support my well-being too, because I felt that others needed these more than I did. Much like a physician is oftentimes the last person to self-refer themselves to get medical attention for an ongoing medical need (which is why they have a reputation for making the worst patients), I was reluctant to ask for help from people and to receive support from any type of service field (i.e. medicine, health coaching, financial planning, legal counsel). At the same time I would highly recommend that my family, my friends, or my clients go to these same specialists -- the doctor, the massage therapist, the chiropractor, the acupuncturist, the therapist, or any other "service provider" when they needed help – I was not taking my own advice.

My pattern is an excellent case study for the Super Hero Syndrome in action. Super Heroes don't think of themselves as heroes, or Super Heroes – they just do what they do and believe that this approach to life is who they are. They don't perceive this way of life as maladaptive; they see nothing wrong with it. They actually think it is all for good – because they continue to get positive reinforcement from the people they are helping (thank yous!) and from others who express appreciation for their kind acts. They can also see the value-add contributions they are making to the world – how their caregiving, parenting, leadership and/or service acts really are making a difference. If no one tells them they should stop, and what they are doing is causing otherwise good (healing) results for others -- why on earth would they want to stop?

This is the most difficult part of Super Hero syndrome; people don't know that they have it because they believe the pattern that they are in is working for them and for those who they are serving. Like an alcoholic that doesn't realize that what began as a simple cocktail has now turned into a series of binge episodes with no end in sight, the Super Hero does not see where their efforts to help (heal) the world shifted into a maladaptive place.

This book will give you further details on why you have these tendencies – which will help you to understand why they are so difficult for you to break. It will also explain how quietly dangerous (scary and risky) these tendencies can be for you, your work, and your quality of life. It is important that you take the discussion seriously in your mind, feel the consequences in your heart, and take action in your body -- because if real positive change is to happen in the world, and if you are the one to do it, then you must be ready. Think of this book as your training tutorial on how to optimize your mind's, heart's and body's capacity – your well-being ultimatum.

Now that I have gone through my own process of making a well-being ultimatum, I can see much more clearly. Like a recovering alcoholic that can re-see past events with a more full, 360 degree perspective – that understands now that what at the time felt good was actually not so good for them or those they care about – I can see now where what I thought was OK (my Super Hero tendencies) really wasn't. In fact, my patterns were dangerous for me, and for those that I care about.

I see now why my Super Hero thinking was well-intended, yet still flawed. My intentions to serve the world – to help as many people as possible in my work and in my life – were not the problem. What was the problem, was that I failed to balance this "call to service" attitude with a commitment to maintaining and restoring my very basic human needs. As humans, we have evolutionary needs for *self-care practices* (to do what is good for us to ensure our longevity) and for *social support* (to share our lives, and to receive help). We don't live as long, or as well, without these two human needs being met. We as individuals, and we as a human race; we have survived this long because we have figured out how to take care of ourselves, and each other.

For most of us humans, the two "S's" are enough most of the time; but not always. Sometimes, when we are faced with a new challenge, we may not have the capacity to handle it alone, or even with support from our social network. In these cases, we need to hire, lean on, and/or contract others who know the way to help us through the difficulty, and to a higher (optimized) level. In this book, I refer to these as *services*, because they may or may not be professional. [Author's Note: I also liked the fact that calling them services means we have a nice-and-easy "3 S" framework here – easy for anyone to remember: self-care, social support and services. And, I use the term services because I think it helps de-stigmatize what it means to "go get help" – we are contracting a service, and that puts us in a place of power. Many folks who need "help" in their life (especially in the area of mental health) don't want to admit it; however, these same people are much more willing to admit they need "services" because it seems more consistent with how they live. The end result is the same – they are receiving expert support as we'll see next].

By services, I mean that we need to rely on the expertise of others to help us to handle tough challenges (stress and/or crisis) and/or to take the next step forward in our evolution (optimize our lived experience). For example, when you hire your hair dresser to rework your hairstyle; when you go to a specialist for that nagging knee problem; when you attend an AA meeting to understand how you can stop drinking; when you attend a toastmaster meeting to learn how to speak in public; when you hire a trainer to help you prepare for your first tri-athalon: you are relying on services. All of these stresses and/or crises have their own "stakes" (some higher than others) but in all cases the human being admits "hey, I need someone who knows what they are doing to help me here".

So, my Super Hero problem was not that my efforts to serve the world were misplaced; with all of its problems, the world needs as many healers as possible (those who live in the service, leadership and/or care of others). The problem was that I failed to recognize that I am a human, and that I need those " 3 S's" – self-care, social support, and services. My commitment to service, my call to lead, and my ability to help others heal took precedence over these basic (3 S) human needs, and in so doing, the basic management of my health, my wellness, my well-being and my life as a whole.

Like the unaware alcoholic, workaholic, or addict, I did not understand that the assumptions I was making (that others needed me more) and my behavior pattern (delaying and/or ignoring these 3 S's) was inherently flawed. My kids came first, closely followed by my work (which I loved) and the rest of my family's needs. Self-care practices, time for support from family and friends (social support) and my use of services to help me manage my finances, my legal privilege, even my hair – could all wait, least until after that particular day's crises were over.

As a smart, educated, functionally healthy, and otherwise happy-with-my-life-and-work person I did not see that this act of putting everything else first was setting myself up for an energy drain (compassion fatigue and burnout, which will be explained in chapter 2). In my mind, at the time, I was just tired, and even exhausted by the fact that the work I was doing was hard; I didn't realize that one of the reasons I was so tired was because I was all outflow (healing efforts) and no inflow. Like any other Mom who gets up with a sick infant at 2 am, I told myself that this was just par for the course (of my life and life in general these days), and that I could push through. I didn't see any of this as maladaptive (bad for me) because I thought that's what was required – by my roles as a mother, a leader, a business owner, and an educator. As the saying goes, "To much who has been given, much is expected."

Here's the funny part, that really isn't funny, and is frankly very hard to admit. What I was doing for my "work" part of the above-mentioned work/life imbalance – is the promotion of health, wellness and well-being. Yes, the work I do, my calling, is to enlighten and empower people about the importance of self-care, social support and the use of health services – in both traditional public health work and also complimentary forms of healthcare (private mind/body medicine and well-being coaching practice). While I built my career training teachers, personal trainers and coaches in promoting self-care education; teaching college courses in health promotion, health policy, exercise physiology and well-being; leading classes and one-on-one sessions in yoga and Pilates; training instructors in these disciplines; and even leading retreats and master classes internationally – I was not always taking my own advice. I spent my days, weeks, months and years training others in the art and science of living well -- to put themselves and their self-care first, to experience peace, and to align their inner reality with their outer -- and I wasn't fully walking that walk myself.

It took a long time for me to come to terms with, and really see, how hypocritical I was in the way that I was living. I would go to bed at night, realizing the day had gone so fast, and I had been so busy encouraging others to be healthy and enlightened, that I had forgotten, and/or ignored my own self-care needs. The keynote that I gave took workout time out of my day; the papers I graded took time out of dinner preparation and fast-food was my answer; my children needed me to drive them to their lesson so my coffee date was rescheduled. Again.

I would close my eyes, telling myself that just for today that this was OK – because this is what this day had asked of me. I would reconcile the hypocratic feelings I felt, by telling myself that these others really needed my time and attention more than my self-care did. I was strong. So my own needs could wait until after the next (fill in the blank here – workshop, manual, or keynote speech) was accomplished. Self-care would wait until after my child's cold was over, or when that next paper was written. That coffee date with my friend could be postponed again, because I had a deadline to meet. My mammogram could wait until next week; it would be too hard to get a sub for my class. I would get to it – to me – eventually.

What I didn't stop to see, which was right under my very eyes, was that every day I had a different story about why my self-care, social support and service needs could wait. Every new day came with its own pressing needs, so despite what I would tell myself there was no magic day that was waiting for me with open arms to engage in a self-care catch-up session.

So most days, the pattern would only repeat itself.

Every day that I put off self-care practices, and didn't ask for help (through social support and/or services), I was becoming more and more of a hypocrite (without intending to be). Interestingly, the word hypocrite derives from a word that the Greeks used to describe a stage actor, who would use a mask while playing a part, to imply the act of pretending or masking. That is exactly what I was doing – masking the fact that I could not reconcile my own self-care needs as a human with my need to "perform" in my work as a health promotion strategist, educator, advocate and healer and in my life as a mom of three.

If you met me or knew me in my real life, you would laugh a bit here, because you would know that I do not normally go walking around my life announcing that I am either a hypocrite or a Super Hero. I am equally embarrassed about both of these ideas. It is even more embarrassing to admit these facts to you here and now.

I come clean with this secret, I take off my mask, to illustrate to you just how sneaky Super Hero syndrome can be, and how dangerous it is too. I share my experiences with you now (and I wrote this book) so that you can learn the warning signs of it. More importantly, I want you to understand the way forward for stopping this pattern of behaviors (this syndrome) if you find you have it too. If someone like me could have it – someone trained as an expert in stress management, alternative therapies, and health promotion -- then it is highly possible that others (not trained in these fields) are susceptible to it too.

By now you may be wondering how I made the ultimate shift – how I made the well-being ultimatum once and for all. It took a pivotal moment for me to see that what I thought was OK (the way I was living) really wasn't. From this place, this bottom, I was able to really turn things around once and for all.

I wish I could say that this pivotal moment came out of my own volition – that I willed it into occurring. But, nothing could be further from the truth. It was only when a crisis occurred (a tsunami of events that traumatized my health, wellness, and well-being) that I started to see these patterns in myself, and to eventually conceptualize them into a behavior pattern, and ultimately a syndrome. The Moment is described in the Prologue of this book.

The details of how I got to this Moment don't ultimately matter, but if you're curious, I'll summarize. In the space of two years my health was threatened by a terminal illness; my life was turned upside down by abusive people who I thought were supportive; my finances were destroyed by a failed business investment -- all while I continued to help the world as a teacher, healer (yoga therapist) and well-being consultant, while I was completing my PhD in health communication, and while I was raising my three children.

If you had met me at this time, you would have most likely only seen the "onstage" performance of my life. You would have seen me as the working single mom, putting herself through a PhD program, and who loved her work in yoga therapy and health and well-being promotion. What you would not have seen, is that "backstage" in my life, I was failing on all fronts. Not only was I trying to handle real-time threats to my financial, physical, and relationship health without help (because I told myself I didn't need these services – that I could just push through); I was also failing to engage in self-care and I certainly wasn't making time for social support (family and friends).

Most of the people I interacted with on a daily basis – clients especially -- had no idea that any of these crises we[...] because I didn't think it was appropriate to share these crise[...] anyone. Just as no one in the Metropolis knows that Super Man is actually Clark Kent, no one knew that Suzie the mom, yoga therapist, professor, and consultant was going through Very Big and Hard Stuff and trying to do it all essentially alone. (I did let a few people in, but only with very deep regret; like a Super Hero that does not want to expose their real identity for fear of losing their 'super power,' I did not want others to know I was having trouble. It wasn't because I was trying to be perfect; it was because I didn't like the attention. I was used to being the one that DID the helping – not the one that RECEIVED it.)

For a long time I quietly accepted the difficult moment at the end of the day, when I would go to bed at night knowing that I had failed my backstage Self. Her need to go for a walk, have coffee with a girlfriend, and/or attend her latest mammogram had been ignored yet again because I had Very Important Work to do. I would start to contemplate how I could snap myself out of the pattern; and sometimes the next day, I would actually do so. But these efforts were generally short-lived, because the minute that Someone Needed Me, I would start thinking like a Super Hero again and would tell myself that my needs could wait until after the day/person/problem was dealt with and/or "saved".

Then one day (described in the prologue to this book), something not big but deeply internal happened. It occurred as I was descending an elevator, heading out to my car, trying to decide what

.ig to plan out how I was going to pull off 6:30 am the next morning when I had a ʌork to check, papers to grade, another paper ɔom to clean. I wondered how I was going to .f while still suffering the effects of an injected meɯ nad numbed my neck while my dermatologist took a large graft ɕ skin (located above my carotid artery) to test a very suspicious-looking mole. As the elevator hit the bottom I did too: I realized that I could no longer keep up the charade. It was time to take off the (Super Hero) mask once and for all.

That day, I made a well-being ultimatum with myself. The moment gave me a new kind of peace that I haven't really lost since. Although it hasn't always been "easy" making the life shifts that I have needed to in order to live in ways that honor both my call to service and my personal (3 S) needs, I do have an internal peace in knowing that I can now honor both. I have learned – in my research, my consulting, and in my own life -- that the best way to optimize well-being is to treat it as a critical process that must be continually cared for, supported, and maintained. Like any recovering addict, I now know that it is only through a daily commitment to my well-being – all parts of it (physical[1], mental, emotional, spiritual and social) and all sides of it (subjective and objective) – that I can truly live the good life in a way that is also good for me (and those I love).

Although I have worked in health promotion since 1997, and have trained at the graduate level in both Health and Kinesiology (MEd) and Health Communication (PhD), it has really been the past four years of my research and my life in which I have been able to come up with an approach to well-being that really *works* -- a well-being ultimatum. I believe the reason why everything finally clicked for me is threefold.

---

[1]When you see the physical kosha/well-being layers discussed throughout this book, please note that my Kosha model of well-being assumes that financial well-being is a sub-construct of physical well-being. Although financial well-being does influence the other Koshas (dimensions of your well-being), I place it here because it influences our ability to function in the world as well as our physical needs being met.

First, while I was going through the process of experiencing, and then recognizing my own compassion fatigue and burnout, I was studying health communication and health promotion at the same time. These studies helped me to recognize what was happening, and gave me the motivation and the resources to research the problem further as a social scientist. Second, my "tsunami" of life experiences forced me to very quickly learn and live the consequences of NOT making a well-being ultimatum. Hitting the wall made me stop and take a good look at how fast I was running – living – and how unsafe it really was. And third, once I put the research and my lived experience together, I was able to see my own faulty patterns with both broad (literature) and deep (personal) perspectives. I was also able to then investigate if this pattern was unique to me, or was not mine alone. I quickly saw in the literature, and in my own client base -- C-suite executives, general officers, corporate leaders, and yes, even yoga teachers – that these same behavior patterns and assumptions were not uncommon. In fact, they were so common I decided to give them a name (Super Hero Syndrome) and to write this book.

The fact that this all happened even as I was continuing to succeed in my career as a health promotion strategist – is both embarrassing and also provided me a wonderful opportunity. Health promotions strategists like me survey a population, find out more about them, and then develop targeted programs (interventions) which support that population in their desired behavior change. So, by identifying the problem I realized I was having as a (social) problem, I was able to design an intervention to address it.

I "test-piloted" it in my own life, and after four years of development, I present to you my findings here, in this book. I delayed sharing this process with the world for a few years because I had to be sure that I wasn't just doing what I always do – helping others before help myself. In recovery programs, you have to be practicing your recovery for a while before you become a leader, or a sponsor. In the yoga community, you have to practice yoga for a long while before you train other instructors. In much the same way, I had to really work my own well-being ultimatum plan, privately, and in small doses with my clients, before the process emerged, and before I could share it.

I should note here that my "test piloting" of this well-being ultimatum process was done in keeping with my work as a health promotion strategist and as a yoga teacher. In medicine and in therapy, it is never acceptable for clinicians to "treat themselves". However, as a yoga teacher, I won't teach a yoga pose that I haven't practiced myself to the point of mastery AND that I haven't learned enough about to understand the consequences of its practice. And, as a health promotion strategists, my work goes a lot better when I fully understand what the population believes to be true – so that I can develop a strategic campaign to address what may be false perceptions as well as behavior change.

Having the condition that this book seeks to address has been embarrassing – both professionally and personally – but has also been my greatest gift. Because I get it.

So ultimately, what you will see in this book is what I have found to be vital components of your well-being ultimatum, gleamed through my own life lessons learned, as well as my research, my work with clients and my overall fascination with what it means to live well. I hope that what has taken me time and sweat to create will actually make it easier for you to optimize your well-being; the healer in me hopes that my personal challenges will not be for naught, and that they can instead be leveraged into your ultimate well-being success.

I should note here that my choice to share some of my personal challenges with regards to my well-being was made to hopefully give others (like you) courage to see how secretly exhausted you are too. By bringing self-care procrastination and/or the never-ending pressure of Super Hero thinking and living behaviors out into the open, I hope to give others the courage to share their stories.

If you are living to serve, heal, and lead others without giving your Self the same courtesy – it is time to see the cold truth that this is draining you, your quality of life, your health, and your ability to be of Service in the first place. It is time for you to see that the people who care about you – both the people you are leading, serving, healing and the people who are in your real (backstage life) – all need for you to get your well-being together. Failure is not an option.

If this discussion resonates with you – because you see yourself in it and/or you know someone who this describes -- this book is for you. If you are a lot like me – you are not just a normal "people pleaser"; you are someone who has a high (and at times extreme) drive towards charity, philanthropy and/or service, this book is dedicated to helping you to make a well-being ultimatum with yourself once and for all.

If you are someone who knows "to those who have been granted much, much is expected," and you take that motto very seriously in the ways that you see yourself and in the ways that you live, then I hope this book helps you to integrate your self-care, your need for social support, and your use of professional services into your to-do list. Although these "3 S" endeavors may not give you the same physiological "high" as helping someone else will, or the same "high" as being of service to the world through your own unique (life) calling, they will ensure that you have enough capacity to meet the demands that these gifts place on you – and the high performance demands you place on yourself in meeting them.

If these themes are resonating with you, but are making you uncomfortable, don't worry. As mentioned before, facing these tendencies is difficult for many reasons. But one way to put your mind at ease through these difficulties is that you should know you really are not alone. I sincerely believe that there are many people out there who are struggling inside with this deep challenge. They don't know about the syndrome; they don't know how many other people are suffering from it; and if they do know (which is doubtful) they don't know where to go to get help for it.

In fact, due to the general lack of awareness surrounding the Super Hero syndrome, I believe it can be considered what my colleagues in health promotion would call a "health disparity". According to the CDC (2015), a health disparity is

> "a preventable difference in the burden of disease, injury, violence, or opportunities to achieve optimal health that are experienced by socially disadvantaged populations. Populations can be defined by factors such as race or ethnicity, gender, education or income, disability, geographic location (e.g., rural or urban), or sexual orientation. Health disparities are inequitable and are directly related to the historical and current unequal distribution of social, political, economic, and environmental resources." (CDC, 2015)

Traditionally, health promotion strategists consider these health disparities to be associated with cultures that are marginalized, or lacking privilege and/or power in some way. (Notice the quote singles out the "disadvantaged".)

It is neither a comfortable, nor comforting thought to consider that we health promotion strategists (and anyone who tries to help the world through their work as a caregiver, leader, parent, healer or serviceworker) who think we are living in lives of advantage are actually disadvantaged in the ways that we are living. Whereas the disadvantaged can't find, access or utilize resources, we Super Heroes have the opposite problem: we believe we don't need resources or that others need them more than we do. Our failure to utilize resources available to us yields us the same result as someone who doesn't know about or who can't access resources: our well-being is less than optimal, or even compromised because we are not using resources that are designed to help us.

Through this book, I seek to illuminate and to addresses this health disparity of healers. Specifically, I hope to help you see something that is actually a little funny if you stop to think about it: you are behaving as though you think you are invincible (like a Super Hero). This is because your failure to access and utilize the "3 S's" implies that you think you are beyond these basic human needs. (This may not be your intention, and in fact you may be an otherwise humble person that would never dream of calling yourself invinsible or a Super Hero – but your behavior is telling this, other story).

The truth is pretty simple. You and I are human. We both need self-care and social support to maintain our longevity (length of our lifetime) and our quality of life (how fun it is while we get to be here). And, at times our life will put us through certain types of events (stresses, or crises), in which we will find ourselves in need of extra (professional) services too. The combination of all three of these 'S's' will help us to optimize both our health and our happiness: our longevity (health status); our physical, mental, social, emotional, and spiritual functioning (wellness); and our quality of life (well-being) are all improved by this powerful, "3 S" combination.

If you really are a Super Hero, about now you are thinking that the idea of the 3 S's (self-care, social support and services) sounds great for other people – but that YOU don't necessarily need all three of them. Or you are wondering how on earth you are supposed to make time for one, two or all three of them, because of course you have _____ to do first.

Of course, that reaction is exactly the problem.

So, although it may be hard to hear the truth, Super Hero, you will indeed need to embrace all three of these 3 S's in order to ensure that your well-being optimized. Take comfort knowing that it's not entirely your fault you are wired to resist this idea; but also take heed knowing that you've got to resist that Super Hero "resistant" lane of thinking enough that you can override it – so you really can make your well-being ultimatum once and for all.

One of the reasons that this line of Super Hero thinking is so hard to delete, amend or transform, is that your hardwiring (physiology) is supporting your current thinking pattern. Physiologically speaking, you really do get a "high" in helping others (as was mentioned earlier in this chapter). Just as your mind/body/heart/spirit feel great when you fall in love, your mind/body/heart/spirit feel great when you are acting in service to others. You also get a second "high" from feeling as though you are accomplishing your sense of "meaning and purpose". People who feel that they are making a real (philanthropic) difference in the world have high well-being; those who identify with being world/change agents love being plugged into their (calling) work. The combination of the feel-good-feelings you get by helping others (engaging in social support) and working to heal the world (engaging in your meaning and purpose) provides a powerful and intoxicating "double shot" of happiness. Combine that shot with another dose of feeling as though society is supporting you – and it is because you are making a difference in the world and you are deemed to be successful at what you do – and you get a three-shot cocktail of joy. You feel happy doing what you are doing; and you have nothing, including your own thoughts, to stop you

As noted earlier, the feel-good-feeling of this dangerous cocktail may feel good at the time but it is not good for you over time. Whether it is because you find yourself having a "hangover" on a short-term basis (needing a retreat or a yoga class to put you back into balance), or you find yourself significantly exhausted and hitting your own personal "bottom" (as is the case in compassion fatigue and burnout), the feel-good-feelings will end eventually. Whether this moment happens because an external series of events brings you to it (as was the case with me) or it happens because you wake up one day realizing you need a deeper sense of balance in your life, you will be really ready make your well-being ultimatum once and for all.

So for you, Super Hero, this book is your own kind of recovery program. It will transform you from an unknowing victim of a quiet health disparity plaguing fellow professionals who work in healing, leading, caregiving and/or service professions, into someone that negotiates between your compelling need to help others and YOUR personal (self-care, social support, and services) needs.

As you make this transformation, and you begin to recognize

and alter your Super Hero thinking, you will become a recovering Super Hero. I affectionately refer to recovering Super Heroes as Strategic Healers. Unlike the Super Hero, the Strategic Healer puts their self-care, their need for social support, and their "maintenance" endeavors (use of services) first. Without question. They do this because they know that this choice strategically optimizes their capabilities – by taking care of themselves they are optimizing their capacity to help others. They also have more energy because they are no longer weighed down by "carrying the weight of the world on their shoulders" and/or the heaviness of their own (Super Hero) masks.

Truth is a lot lighter, and more free, than being perfect all of the time.

My objectives in writing this book for you, are therefore threefold. First, I hope that the book (and the process of creating your well-being ultimatum) will inspire you to engage in self-care practices daily that enhance your health, well-being, relationships and quality of life. Second, I hope that in making this well-being ultimatum, that you will no longer be afraid or reluctant to ask for help (social support) when you need it. And third, I hope that you will not hesitate to actually utilize whatever services are necessary (both within healthcare, alternative medicine and/or within your community) to ensure that all aspects of your health, wellness and well-being are managed and protected. A fourth, bonus objective, is that I hope that this process will transform you from someone who is an unknowing Super Hero into a Strategic Healer advocate – one who encourages other Super Heroes to transform into Strategic Healers by your own lived example.

If you still have doubts, don't worry. Rest assured that this process will not ask you to give up your compelling need to help, lead, serve, teach, or heal others. It will not ask you to give up your "cape" (your call to help the world). It will not make the pace of your life slow down. However, it will ask you to take off that cape too as needed to ensure your well-being is truly optimized (subjectively and objectively) and in all dimensions (physical, social, mental, spiritual and emotional).

As noted above, future chapters will give you the information you need to tackle the creation of your well-being ultimatum head on. Chapter two will give a brief overview of the science of stress, crisis, compassion fatigue and burnout, so that you can better understand why it is so important that you take care of your 'stress management' (3 S) needs. Chapter three will unpack the science of well-being, and why both personal (self-rated) appraisals and objective (other-based) appraisals are key to ensuring that your well-being plan not only feels good to you but is also good for all dimensions of you. Chapter four will unpack the dimensions of your well-being, by using the Kosha framework – I use the ancient yogic and Ayurvedic system of the koshas to explain why and how it's important for all dimensions of your well-being to get along.

With this background information, as well as the call to action that I hope this chapter provides for you, I then take you through a strategic planning process which will help you to create your well-being ultimatum. In Chapter 5, you will create a vision statement which will articulate what you ultimately hope to give to the world. You will create a mission statement which will explain how you will go about achieving that vision in your own unique way. You will conduct a stakeholder analysis with yourself – you will ask all of the roles that you play every day to have a "meeting" and to discuss, negotiate, and compromise on a way forward that makes sense for your mission and your vision. You will also conduct a stakeholder analysis of the people in your life who represent the various dimensions of your health, wellness and well-being that are especially important to you.

If you are unfamiliar with stakeholder analyses don't worry; this is an easy process of surveying key people who have a "stake" in your success. Most stakeholder analyses ask you to focus on the people who influence your mission. For a company, this may be a survey of customers, investors, board members, and employees. The findings are then collected together to determine a way forward that makes the best sense for all and which aligns to your vision, mission and goals.

Your external stakeholder analysis will similarly ask you to interview people that you deem to be representative of the "company" that is you and your life. The list may include (but is not necessarily limited to) your doctor, your lawyer, your best friend, your spouse, your child, your parents, your personal trainer, your employees, and your team members. The strategic planning process will help to illuminate who should be on this list, and it will be up to you to ensure that all of their perspectives are captured and heard. Stakeholder analyses only really work when we really listen to what our stakeholders have to really say.

Your internal stakeholder analysis will ask you to interview a different kind of subcommittee – the various dimensions of your Self. I like to think of these "dimensions of you" as "role identities" in your life; your internal stakeholder analysis will ask you to get to know these roles, to learn what they find important, and to get them to negotiate with each other as needed in order for you to optimize your well-being over the short-term and the long-term.

This approach of "role identity negotiation" sounds a little New-Agey (and is reminiscent of Archetypes by Jung) but is actually inspired by the "role identity" work of Ting-Toomey (1999); and the role identity negotiation work of Jackson (2002) and Collier (2005; 2009). It takes their work in a different direction though. As intercultural communication scholars, their work tends to place "role identities that we play" into cultural contexts; to learn why there may or may not be discordant beliefs between the expectations of people or groups in a communicative interchange.

I apply their work in a different way – helping people to conceptualize the wellness and well-being dimensions of their life as "roles" too. By approaching our need for work/life balance by recognizing the different roles we play in both work and life – as mother, as father, as worker, as server, as teacher, as healer, as leader, as friend, as family member, as caregiver – we can start to realize that there are bound to be times when our lives will feel out of balance because of competing (role) demands. Just as every individual that works for a company has a different idea of what is and what is not "good" for the company over time, so too do each of your different "roles" have sometimes different (and even conflicting) ideas of what is best for you. It is little wonder therefore that at times our work/life balance is out of balance; we have many different dimensions (roles) within us that are all trying to have a voice in your well-being.

So, your well-being ultimatum will ask you to conduct an internal stakeholder of these role needs. Specifically, you will be asked to get to know each of the "roles" you play in your life, and to imagine that each of them is being called to a strategic planning meeting in which they will "negotiate" your overall well-being. It is an exercise in your imagination of course, but this particular piece of the well-being ultimatum process has proven to be very illuminating for every client I have ever worked with – including and especially myself.

The combination of these external and internal stakeholder analyses will provide you with both subjective perspectives (your own) and objective perspectives (from the people that are important to you) of your well-being. This approach is unique (and more time-intensive) to most health coaching processes, which generally does not ask you to go and secure additional data from the people in your life and/or to unpack your inner role identities and their assumptions for your well-being.

I ask you to take on this longer road (of conducting data

collection) rather than simply writing down your goals as you see them right now, because I want to make sure that you have a full view of any underlying problems and barriers to your well-being. If the many roles you play every can't get along, how on earth can you live in authenticity or equanimity – and optimize your well-being?

I also have you go through this (longer) process for creating your well-being strategic plan (ultimatum), because I want you to have the benefit of both subjective and objective perspectives of your well-being. By engaging in both internal (role) and external (support team) stakeholder analyses, you will gain a 360 degree (subjective and objective) view of your life. This viewpoint will ensure that your well-being ultimatum plan really is designed and followed in ways that protect your life (longevity and quality) interests.

The next step in your well-being ultimatum process, after vision and mission statement design and stakeholder analyses, will be a SWOT analysis. This type of assessment asks you to come clean with yourself and boil down what you have discovered thus far into four categories: "Strengths, Weaknesses, Opportunities and Threats" (SWOT). This is similar to a navigation process when you are going on a trip: you decide where you want to be (vision), you decide why you want to go and what is important to you in terms of the experience of getting there (mission). Then, the real preparation starts when you assess what resources you have (within your own capabilities as well as external resources) that are available to you that you can employ to get from here to there in the way that you want to. The "SWOT" component simply helps you to be honest with yourself in terms of what is and is not available to you on this journey – and helps you to anticipate challenges (weaknesses and threats) as much as you celebrate your success (strengths and opportunities).

Your well-being ultimatum process will therefore help you to boil down your current SWOT "reality" so that you can see an honest and realistic way forward for optimizing your well-being going forward. You will specify and outline the types of self-care, social support, and services you will need in order to maximize your strengths and opportunities, and minimize your threats and weaknesses. You will create a contract that summarizes this outline, and you will be ask someone else in your life – someone you respect and trust – to sign your contract with you. This person could be a buddy, or a coach; the process can also be used by mental health clinicians as long as it is in keeping with their particular training and standards of professional conduct. (Although I train coaches in my system, I don't copyright it; I hope it is helpful to as many people as possible).

You will notice that throughout this strategic planning process – from mission and vision statement design, to SWOT analysis, to stakeholder inquiry – you will be asked to document your process as well as your key aims. The combined process will enable you to both monitor and evaluate your efforts – which are critical for both motivation to continue and adherence to the entire ultimatum plan. By monitoring and evaluating your success on a regular basis, you will be much less likely to fall off of the (well-being) wagon, and you will be better able to track the benefits of the changes you are making over time. (Please see the assessment tools for evaluating your well-being on my website: www.drsuziecarmack.com).

Through this comprehensive strategic planning process – from vision, to mission, to stakeholder analyses (both internal and external) to SWOT analysis, to daily/weekly/annual contractual plan, buddy system and to evaluation – you will ensure that the paradigm-level shift of your life that you have been seeking really does occur. As you can see, we aren't focusing on what a strategist would call tactics or what a social marketing specialist would call behavior change – another diet, another set of tips for cutting out fat, another program for exercise. Instead, we are taking a much more comprehensive and strategic approach to analyzing and improving the ways that you perceive, evaluate, experience, and engage with your life. The ultimate goal of this approach is to not only support behavior change (as needed for your well-being optimization) but to also optimize both your well-being literacy and your lived experience of well-being – to optimize your ability to live well in ways that are good for you.

It is my ultimate hope that you will come to realize that your ability to perform like a Super Hero (help, serve and/or lead in the world) will only be optimized if you are willing to make a daily (self-care), weekly (social support) and monthly (services) commitment to your Self. You will know that your ability to save the world is compromised if you procrastinate these "3 S" needs for even one more day. You will know that you are of no use to anyone if you aren't here in the world in the first place – and the only way for you to stick around here a little longer in the world is by maintaining these needs in ways that empower you. You will know that you have no choice but to make this ultimatum, because the thought of letting yourself, or anyone you lead, care for, serve, and/or heal down is too much to bear. These paradigm-level shifts in assumptions will enable you to optimize your well-being subjectively and objectively; they will shift not only your behavior, but your lived experience of "the good life".

For all of these reasons, I call this a Well-Being Ultimatum – because your quality of your life, and your longevity, really will not wait one more day. According to Merriam-Webster, an "ultimatum" is:

> "a final offer or demand made by one party to another, especially in diplomatic negotiations, expressing or implying the threat of serious consequences or the breakoff of relations if the terms are not accepted." (Merriam-Webster, 2015).

By this definition, the demand you are making is with yourself. The diplomatic negotiations you will be making are between your compelling need to help others (i.e. heal, lead, serve and/or teach) and your own personal, human needs for self-care, social support, and services (external resources). If you are indeed a Super Hero, you are most likely not negotiating between your Call to Service and your "3 S" needs – but you shouldn't be. In fact, serious consequences can occur for both the length and the quality of your life if this negotiation does not begin immediately. Your evolution depends on your ability to put the 3 S's first – even when the day tells you otherwise.

Hence, the time has come for you to see that there is indeed an implied threat, and serious consequences if the terms of such a negotiation (between your self-care, social support, resource/service and call to heal) are not accepted. This threat is expressed every time – every day – that you forgo your own self-care needs to help and heal others. The consequences are felt by both the quality of your life (on a day-day basis and over time) and by the quantity of your life (your longevity).

The minimum consequence that you face if you do not make this well-being ultimatum, is that your well-being is not optimized; you will not be living as well as you otherwise could have. The maximum consequence you face if you do not make this well-being ultimatum, is that your longevity will be threatened; you will not live as long as you otherwise would have because the 3 S's are all forms of preventative health that enhance your longevity. The irony is that either of these consequences (i.e. not living well enough and/or long enough) will get in the way of what you have wanted to do all along – heal others – in one way or the other.

So, yes, it is time that you make your well-being ultimatum – an ongoing commitment to the recovery of your well-being (quality of life) and longevity (quantity of life). Do it for you. Do it for your inner Super Hero. Do it for all of the people you help with the important work that you do. Do it for your physiology so that all of your systems can optimally handle your day-day stress and the major life crises and work/life balance issues that occur for you. Do it for your sister, your son, or your grandmother, so that you can lead them by your example. Do it when no one is watching, and when everyone is watching. Just do it.

Make no mistake. Once you decide to make the commitment to your well-being ultimatum, you will have a lot of work to do. And, like any recovery program, this well-being ultimatum will be tough in quiet ways on a daily basis that in many cases no one will see except for you. As stated previously, it will require you to engage in "diplomatic negotiations" between your self-care needs and the compelling need you have to serve, lead and heal others. Like a recovering addict who must decide – in a tempting instant -- between the immediate gratification of "just one drink" and the long-term gratification that comes with a daily commitment to recovery, you will have tempting instants too. That addict must decide in the moment between the high of getting high, and the high of living well and preventing the "serious life consequences" that come with substance abuse from occurring. You too must decide between the immediate highs you receive from putting others first and the long-term protection and gratification of putting yourself first – and the consequences that accompany either of these choices. I want you to see every decision to procrastinate your 3 S's as this "just one" decision.

This process of negotiating between your short term well-being (i.e. the physiological "boost" you get from helping others) and your long-term well-being (i.e. your comprehensive well-being and longevity) will require that you rewire some of your thought patterns. It will ask you to hold yourself accountable to your self-care, even when it's messy (and you have to say no to someone, thing, or group in the world). It will shift the power at the bargaining and negotiation table, from the part of you that heals others, to the part of you that knows that self-care and the willingness to lean on others (social support and services) comes first. Period.

I will caution you here that the last part – asking others for help – is often times the hardest part for any Super Hero. It's not surprising when you consider that in the comics, the only people who have helpers are the villains.

There is one exception to this rule: one Super Hero that asks for help. Batman. So if it helps you to take the edge off of the difficulties that you face in making this well-being ultimatum, you can decide that you want to be like him. Like Batman, you will need to make time to retreat to the lair of your self-care, so that you can recharge (like he did with the Batmobile, a key symbol of his power). Like Batman, you may need to allow others to serve you (like he did when he allowed his butler to fix his car). Like Batman, you may even ask for help when you are out of the lair of your self-care, serving and saving the world (like he did when he accepted Robin's assistance). And, like Batman, you may need to lean on other services for help (like he did when he and the Commissioner collaborated to rid the Metropolis of the bad guys).

You may be laughing at this analogy – but it's actually not funny. Most Super Heroes like you, are really uncomfortable with the lair (self-care), and/or are uncomfortable with receiving help from others who are close to them (social support) or from experts (services).

The other bit of hard news – which you should know before you read further – is that the process will be ongoing, long after the book is over for you. Becoming a Strategic Healer does not mean that we get to a place where we never have to work through this juggling act between our desire to serve and our self-care needs. On the contrary, it means that we are willing to be as honest with ourselves as we ask others to be in order to help them. It means that we've got to do the hard work ourselves, so that we can continue to learn, live and grow. If it helps to know, I am doing it too. Even as I write this book, I am balancing my self-care, reaching out for help, and receiving the support of services despite how uncomfortable all three of these sometimes make me feel.

Here's the best, and most freeing news of all: when you make this well-being ultimatum, you will feel a lot more free and energetic. That dynamic energy will help you to experience life in a deeper and heart-felt way, and will also give you more energy to do the very work you can't stop yourself from doing: service, leadership and healing. If this book has gotten to you a little late – you are already in a health crisis and/or your well-being is burned out or fatigued – it will help you to find your way back to feeling yourself again.

So don't worry. You are a Super Hero after all; you can handle hard work. Take that energy you give so willing to helping, leading, serving and healing others, and throw some in your own direction. Apply that same tenacity you have to helping others, into the commitment to your self-care, so that when the negotiations between your self-care and your Super Hero get tough – and they will – that you (your well-being and your longevity) will always win. When you put your mind to helping others, there is nothing stopping you; why not put your mind to helping your Self too?

The truth is, that I am excited for you. Because when you decide to make and follow-through on this mandate, this well-being ultimatum -- you will see an immediate improvement in the quality and the quantity of your life. Underneath the surface of your skin, your physiologic capacity to handle anything life throws at you (including day-day stress, difficult life events, and your compelling need to serve) will increase. This improved capacity will prevent, or manage compassion fatigue or burnout – exhausting conditions which plague Super Heroes that do not commit to self-care. Your health prognosis may even improve, because your self-care has many preventative health benefits. And, when you make and follow-through on your well-being ultimatum, your optimized health will enable you to be an even better super hero. Not only will you be able to do the work that you are compelled to do (to help, heal, lead or serve others); your behavior and lifestyle will quietly give others the courage to do the same for themselves.

At the end of the day, the world does not need another burned out Super Hero; it needs compassionate humans who have the strength to help each other back to peace, and still have enough energy left to enjoy their lives. We can only be of service to others, if we are willing to do the hard work ourselves – and that includes asking for help and making our health, wellness and well-being priority one. Our own strategic healing process is ongoing, and must be. For if we fail to honor the needs of our body, mind, heart and life, we will undermine the capacity we have to make a difference in the world.

So take off your cape, roll up your sleeves and open your mind and heart. Because it's time for you to get your life back.

CHAPTER 2
KRYPTONITE: WHY STRESS, COMPASSION FATIGUE AND BURNOUT FOSTER ILL-BEING AND THREATEN YOUR WELL-BEING

In the first chapter, we discussed why Super Heroes like you may need to make a Well-Being Ultimatum. I explained how those of us who spend our time healing the world -- as leaders, clinicians, teachers, Service members and/or practitioners – have human needs too. When we do balance our "Super Hero" drive to serve our calling in the world, with the 3 S's (self-care, social support and services), we become "strategic healers". But if we don't balance the outflow of our Super Hero-ness with the inflow that we get from the 3 S's, compassion fatigue and/or burnout are likely to result.

So, why is that?

In order to understand what compassion fatigue and burnout really are, and why they can so easily plague healers, we've got to understand the science of stress, and the science of well-being. This chapter will therefore explain the science of stress (in a very quick, high-level way) and the next two chapters will unpack the science of well-being. Together, these chapters will give you a full understanding of how healers are so vulnerable to compassion fatigue and burnout, and why well-being ultimatums are in order for those healers who are trying to prevent, or mange these conditions.

Most people cringe when they hear the word stress. The very word that describes what it feels like to be out of balance (have stress) can cause you to feel even more out of balance, because it reminds you of what it feels like to be out of balance. Simply put, thinking about stress can create the feeling of stress.

As noted by an article in *Psychology Today* (2010), your perception and/or experience of stress is actually based on your assumptions about a situation (stressful event) and not on the situation itself. In other words, if we believe that an event (a stressor) is bad for us, it will be. Our entire system is rigged to react to this stressor in a way that seeks to either remove ourselves from it (fly); get rid of it (fight) or ignore it and hope for it to pass (freeze).

However, if we believe an event is not bad for us (we have adapted to it), it won't be stressful (i.e. it won't create a stress-based response). Our experience, our perceptions, our beliefs and our assumptions about an event come together in a way that can "make or break" that experience as something that deserves the "all points bulletin" of a stress response (or not). You might conceptualize this as a "surprise" – if you know something is coming and/or what to do about it, it is less surprising. Stress is similar in that if we know something is coming and/or what to do about, it is "less stressful."

If you encounter a moment, a life event, or an experience as something that is familiar, and that familiarity gives you "no cause for concern" then your stress response will be diminished, or may not even kick in in the first place. If however, you encounter a moment, a life event, or an experience as something that is not familiar – a surprise – then your sympathetic response will kick in and your physiologic abilities to flee, fight and/or freeze will go into high alert.

In the high alert example, your physiology will signal all of your systems to secret the hormones and functions that you need to enact your reaction – your heart will start pounding faster; your digestive processes will slow/stop; your pupils will dilate. Whether you actually move away from the "surprise" (stress) or not; whether you freeze in fear or not; and whether you try to fight/destroy the surprise in some way or not – your body will have a physiological reaction that will prepare you for these endeavors. In other words, your physiology won't know the difference if these activities actually occurred. For example, your heart will begin pumping faster to support your ability to run away from the stress; your heart rate will continue at an accelerated pace even if you decide not to actually run away.

As you can see, your "fight, flight or freeze" stress response is a full systems alert: all of your major physiological systems have similar responses to the one just mentioned (for your heart).

What is interesting about us humans, is that it really isn't the stressor itself that creates this stress response. It's (1) whether or not your mind/body perceives the stress as being an "alerting surprise" – something new it hasn't dealt with before and/or (2) something that you find yourself needing to rally for in order to address. Just because one man or woman perceives an event to be a surprise (stressful), does not mean that another man or woman may have the same (surprise) reaction.

Like beauty, stress is in the eye of the beholder.

To make things even more interesting when we think about this ability that you have to respond to a stress (surprise), is that your body doesn't know the difference between a "good" surprise (stress) and a "bad" one. This is why you felt as much of a rush of adrenaline in the fearful moment that someone startled you by coming around a corner unexpectedly, as you did when you saw someone you instantly fell in love with for the first time and you weren't sure if you should run towards them, away from them, or stay put for lack of knowing what to do with the overwhelming feelings you are experiencing. Although the first example is based in fear, and the second one is based in love, both of these surprising (stressful) moments results in physiologically identical "stress" responses.

Counter to this "fight, flee or freeze" stress response which is enacted by your sympathetic nervous system, is the "rest and digest" system of your parasympathetic system. If you believe that you are not susceptible to stress (because you feel safe, secure and are not "surprised" by a moment, life event or experience) and/or you do not feel you need to "ramp up" and "rally" your capabilities in order to respond to an event, then your body will be able to flip out of the "stress response" and into this parasympathetic, or "rest and digest response".

It is important to note that the sympathetic (fight/flight/flee) response is the one we live in most of the time, and for good reason. We have evolved as humans because we have the human capacity to adjust to threats. If our physiology decided to take random breaks (in the rest and digest mode), we would find ourselves in vulnerable places that would not ensure our longevity -- as individuals and as a species.

But even though we spend most of our time in this "readiness state" – ready to fly, flee or fight in order to adapt to the stress/surprise -- that doesn't mean that this is good for us over time. We were actually "designed" as humans to have more of a balance between our time spent in the sympathetic response, and the parasympathetic response than most of us do today. Much like a lion has bouts of running after prey, running from threats, and lying lazily in the field under a tree – we were designed to balance our sympathetic needs with parasympathetic ones. Our health, and our well-being is compromised when we do not allow ourselves a sufficient balance between these two systems.

The diagram on the next page depicts your sympathetic and parasympathetic systems, and illustrates how each system has a team of responses that enables you to either "fight/fly/flee" (yang) or "rest/digest and breed" (yin).

Just like your physiology will adapt to a run over time in ways that alter your mental, physical and social capacity, your physiology can also adapt to life events and situations over time as well. Your

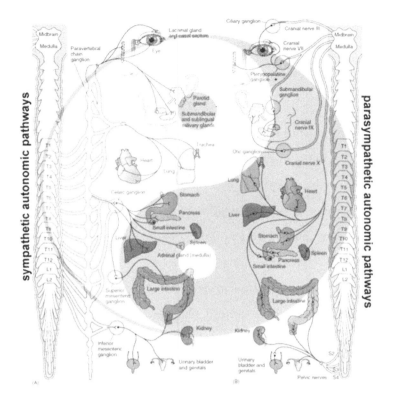

Source: Stroka (2015)

physiology adapts to the life events that you want to happen, and to the ones that you don't want to happen.

Recent research in the area of health psychology has taken this understanding of stress a step further. We have known for a long time that we respond to stress with either our sympathetic or parasympathetic response systems. New research has also found that if we believe that the experiences of "stress" is bad for us over time, it will be. If we believe that stress is actually an opportunity for our minds and bodies to adapt and/or become resilient, then stress does not have as many negative effects on our health, well-being and longevity. Recent studies have shown that people who think stress is bad for them over time have a higher mortality rate (die sooner) than those who think that stress is essentially their friend (McGonigal, 2015).

Putting this all together, you can see why stress management is not about "ridding your life" of stress. It would be naïve to think that you will never be surprised by a moment, life experience or situation again. Instead, stress management begins with accepting that although we are hard-wired to fight, flee, or freeze in response to any new stressor, we can manage ourselves during the moment we experience the surprise. We can decide if we will continue to treat the stressor as something we should fear, and continue trying to avoid, destroy or ignore (i.e. we can decide if we will stay in the conventional "stress response"). Or, we can choose to adapt to the stress, by deciding that the stressor is an opportunity for us to become stronger: the stress is greeted as a catalyst for us to adapt and change (improve our resiliency) over time.

Simply put – the next time you find yourself being surprised by life, by something that you wanted to happen or something that you didn't want to happen, notice if your first response is to fight it, flee from it or freeze in fear over it. If so, choose to override that response by "digesting it" or "resting with it" by making friends with it.

By making the decision to "make friends with stress" we can further ease the physiologic challenges that stress puts on our human (homeostatic) system, and we can also make a positive difference in the longevity and quality of our lives.

About now you are probably wondering, "how exactly can I make friends with stress?" And, where do compassion fatigue and burnout fit in?

We're getting there.

I'll begin by saying that it isn't easy to make friends with stress. But the following suggestions are drawn from the assumptions I make in my own life when I face stress (good and bad stress), and is also the same guidance I have given to clients over the years. It is a set of assumptions that has evolved over time; but it has not been scientifically measured or examined in great detail (at least not to my knowledge). I invite you to see if this approach works for you as it has for many of my clients.

Your ability to adapt to stress – both good stress and bad stress – is related to (and possible dependent upon) your inner and external capacities.

I define your *inner capacity* as a combination of four things: (1) your self-efficacy (whether you believe you can do something); (2) your experiences thus far (whether you have actually handled the stress previously); (3) your self-concept (what you believe to be true about yourself) and (4) your "locus of control" – how much power you believe you have to direct the course and experience of your life. All four of these dimensions of your inner capacity work together, as a team, to help you to deal with stressors all day long -- usually without your even knowing about it. Your inner capacity is working behind the scenes (within you) to help you feel less stressed about the stimuli (stressors) that you face all day long.

Stressors that are familiar to your body, your mind, and/or your lifestyle do not feel stressful, because your inner capacity knows how to handle them. You might say they "see the stress coming." This is because once your mind (mental capacity), body (physical capacity), and/or heart (emotional capacity) adapt to a stress, this inner capacity knows what to do.

Your adaptation to the stress occurs because you believe you are capable (i.e. you have high self-efficacy for dealing with the stress); you have handled something similar (i.e. you have experience dealing with the stress or a similar one); you believe in your Self and your abilities (i.e. you have high self-concept) and/or you believe you have control over what occurs (i.e. you feel you can direct the stressful event to a favorable outcome). You think you could handle it (self-efficacy), you have handled it (experience), you can handle it (self-concept) and you are optimistic that you will handle it (control). Most of the time, this all happens without your actually thinking about it – hence the term inner capacity.

Your ability to adapt to stress is not only supported and enhanced by these four dimensions of your inner capacity, it is also reinforced and supplemented by your *external capacity*. My definition of external capacity has two components: (1) tools (including services and other resources) and (2) a team (people). Research has shown that people who have strong social support (a good partner and/or team) and/or feel that they can rely on services (medical, community, or other programs) have higher well-being. To use a phrase used in law enforcement, your external capacity is your "backup" – it reinforces and supports what you can do in the same way that one officer's skillset reinforces and supports another's on a call.

Together, inner capacity and external capacity help you to manage, ameliorate and adapt to the experience of stress. They work in tandem like guards. By helping you to 'fight' (manage, ameliorate and/or adapt to) stress, they protect and optimize your well-being. Together they remind you that you are strong enough to handle (manage) stress, and that even in this strength, it is OK to lean on others for help.

Where this approach to inner and external stress management capacity can be helpful, is not when these capacities are working well and are functional; when things are "easy" for us in terms of stress management we may even forget about them. Instead, where they are actually more helpful is when we find ourselves in "times of trouble" – stress and/or crisis.

In a real life, tough, moment that pushes us to our edge, it is helpful to unpack whether or not we feel our inner capacity and/or our external capacity is compromised. Maybe the feeling of being pushed to our edge is happening because we aren't sure if we can take on the stress (i.e. have low self-efficacy). Maybe it is because we have not had experience with something similar; we don't know if we are strong enough and/or we don't know if we have the power to direct an outcome that we hope for. All of these fears speak to our perceived diminished inner capacity to handle the stressful event.

In much the same way, compromises to our external capacity can also leave us overwhelmed by stress. If we don't allow ourselves to ask for "back-up" – either by leaning on others for support (team) and/or for expertise and services (tools), then we can easily become overwhelmed trying to do it all ourselves.

This feeling of being overwhelmed by stress creates the experience of ill-being – the opposite of well-being. It therefore diminishes our ability to optimize our well-being; if we are overwhelmed by stress, then our well-being is compromised.

As noted in chapter 1, this is the fundamental issue with Super Heroes – although they generally have high inner capacities they often fail to build and/or utilize their external capacity. This creates a scenario that can manifest ill-being, and threaten the optimization of their well-being as well as their ability to serve the world.

And this is one of the reasons that I wrote this book. It has been my experience that people who are hard-wired to think like a Super Hero (see Chapter 1) do not take the advice to improve and enhance their inner and/or external capacity easily. More often that not, it takes a moment in which "the universe" gives them a mandate of some kind. Whether it is a call-to-action from a friend, a health scare, or a financial crisis, the time comes when they realize they can no longer ignore their external capacity needs. They realize they can't do it alone. They realize they need back-up.

Leading up to this moment, there are often warning signs that indicate their well-being is in question or at least not optimal. Sometimes people see these warnings, before the "universe" forces them to address the (stress) issue. Other times they don't.

Allow me to explain what I now know to be warning signs, that I wish someone had told me about several years ago – before I had my own well-being crisis.

In scholarship, we actually have "formal" (evidence-based) names for these warning signs (syndromes), and they come in two seemingly similar, but actually unique types. The clinical condition (secondary stress disorder) of Compassion Fatigue is one, and Burnout is the other.

Like their names imply, both Compassion Fatigue and Burnout feel draining – but in different ways. Compassion Fatigue makes us wonder "Where did my energy go?" and "Why can't I push through this?". We find meaning in what we are doing (i.e. healing work), but we feel we don't have enough energy to take it on or perform to our full capacity. We quietly hope the feeling of being drained will disappear at some point if we just push through a little longer, a little harder. We keep chasing our well-being – and exhaust ourselves the more we try to catch it.

Compassion Fatigue has been described in the *Medical Dictionary* (2009) as "cynicism, emotional exhaustion, or self-centeredness occurring in a health care professional previously dedicated to his or her work and clients". It has also been described as "the continuing stress of meeting the often overwhelming needs of patients and their families" when discussed in nursing contexts (Lombardo & Eyre, 2011). Both of these descriptions, as well as others, illustrate the overwhelming nature of Compassion Fatigue.

Author Patricia Smith, a leading expert in the field of Compassion Fatigue, has developed an assessment protocol to test individuals for Compassion Fatigue. (See her website compassionfatigue.org for resources). Her work emphasizes the importance of self-care practices, as well as social support, in the prevention and/or healing of compassion fatigue. As she notes on her website:

> "When caregivers focus on others without practicing self-care, destructive behaviors can surface. Apathy, isolation, bottled up emotions and substance abuse head a long list of symptoms associated with the secondary traumatic stress disorder now labeled: Compassion Fatigue" (Smith, 2015)

When considered from a capacity perspective, Compassion Fatigue is an issue of one's inner capacity being overly emphasized and one's external capacity being underutilized.

The individual may have the belief (self-efficacy) to help, lead and/or serve others; experience in doing so, belief in themselves and even believe that they can somehow control a difficult (healing) outcome; however, they do not allow themselves to rely on external capacity resources (teams and/or tools) in ways that adequately support and protect these efforts. The result is that the person feels as though the "weight of the world is on their shoulders" -- and it is. They are relying on their inner capacity without relying on other world-based (external) resources for additional support in order to handle stress: both the stress that comes from their healing work, and the everyday stresses they experience as a human.

At some point, the world becomes too heavy relative to the inner capacity strength of this Super Hero. Compassion Fatigue is the result.

Burnout is a more existential problem than Compassion Fatigue: it makes us wonder "Why am I doing this to myself?" If Compassion Fatigue is about the world feeling heavy on our shoulders, then Burnout is about putting the world down – and wondering why we were holding it in the first place.

Burnout is described as "the condition of someone who has become very physically and emotionally tired after doing a difficult job for a long time." (*Merriam-Webster*, 2015). It therefore may bring a deeper sense of exhaustion than Compassion Fatigue – much like a "bottom" moment feels a lot deeper and bigger for an addict than a hangover.

Most of the measures of Burnout examine issues surrounding Engagement; in fact, Burnout and Engagement are considered as being (almost) polar opposites of each other much like Depression and Happiness are viewed as being (almost) polar opposites. Burnout can even be understood as a form of Depression; it can bring with it a detachment from everything including the things that used to bring us joy. (Author's Note: if you are experiencing a feeling of being "drained" you should have a clinician administer a Depression screen as well as Compassion Fatigue and Burnout screenings to diagnose whether or not your experience is resulting from Depression, Compassion Fatigue, Burnout, or something else. If you are having serious thoughts about any form of harm or self-harm, call 911 immediately).

In my experience, Super Heroes are as vulnerable to Burnout as they are to Compassion Fatigue. Although they can present in similar ways at a surface level – Compassion Fatigue is an imbalance issue, while Burnout is is an endurance issue. In Compassion Fatigue, the individual is overly relying on their inner capacity relative to their external capacity. In Burnout, inner and/or external capacities have become short-circuited and/or exhausted over time. The solution for the Super Hero with either Compassion Fatigue or Burnout is the same: they need to take time to restore their energy balance (of inflow and outflow) and/or they need to look to new resources for replenishment, revitalization and/or support.

It has been my experience that more often than not, most Super Heroes do not know that they are suffering from Compassion Fatigue or Burnout. They are too busy helping others, until a situation "forces" them to take a deeper look at why they are feeling tired, overwhelmed, and/or drained.

Whether it is the energy imbalance issue of Compassion Fatigue (which results from too much outflow relative to inflow) or the energy endurance issue of Burnout (which results from too much performance demand on existing inner and external capacities), the result is the same. The Super Hero no longer has well-being, because they are physically, mentally, emotionally, socially and even spiritually drained. Their inner and external capacities are not being utilized in ways that can optimally handle stress and optimize well-being.

Putting it all together: here's why stress, compassion fatigue and burnout must be addressed by Super Heroes like you. The work you do is stressful – even if you view it as good stress, it still takes a toll on your mind, your body and your life. If you don't take time for the 3 S's (self-care, social support and services) then you will be more likely for stress to overwhelm you in the form of Compassion Fatigue and/or Burnout.

So if you're going to be a healer in the world, you've got to be strategic about it. The world needs Super Heroes who are well-equipped, and optimized, to handle their life stresses and the stressful work that they do. The world needs teachers who aren't so tired that they can't teach; leaders who aren't so exhausted that they can't lead; parents who aren't so depleted that they can't parent; clincians who aren't so ill that they can't heal; military members who aren't so stressed that they can't serve. These healers' important, life-changing and healing work is compromised if the very person delivering these services – the Super Hero -- can no longer accomplish their healing / calling because they are drained by Compassion Fatigue and/or Burnout.

We need Super Heroes to not be overwhelmed by stress; we can't have them falling victim to the Kryptonite of thinking that they don't need to restore and renew their inner and external capacities. We really need these Super Heroes to instead optimize their well-being by optimizing their inner and external capacities – and in so doing their well-being.

If we really are going to have a better, safer, more healthy world, then we've got to start by taking care of our Super Heroes – including and especially you.

And that is why in chapter 1, I explained that this book is dedicated to helping you to better understand and manage your well-being once and for all. By making efforts to build and manage your inner and external capacities (which are foundational components of this well-being ultimatum) you can both manage the negative effects of long-term stress, and optimize your well-being. You will be better equipped – internally and externally – to handle the stressful demands of your (healing) work, and your high stakes life. And the world will benefit from a more optimal, healthy, and happy you.

You will notice that the fundamental suggestion I make throughout this book -- that Super Heroes need self-care, social support, and services just like the everybody else – is essentially an easy-to-adapt framework for building your inner and external capacities. All three of these "S's" will help you to improve your stress balance (i.e. take temporary reprieves in the parasympathetic land of 'rest and digest') as well as your stress response (i.e. optimize your ability to 'fight, flee or freeze' as you need to in your Super Hero work and in your life).

You will see that in Chapter 5, I will walk you through a specific process of determining which self-care, social support, and service needs may be right for you. But before we go there, I would like to first unpack for you the science of well-being. In chapter 3, we will examine the surprisingly complex and at times confusing landscape of well-being science, and you will learn why both subjective and objective analyses of well-being are important for writing your whole well-being story. In chapter 4, we will unpack the major dimensions (types) of your well-being by using a framework I developed based on the Kosha system of yoga.

Together, these two chapters will help you to have a more informed perspective of the "sides" of your well-being (subjective and objective) and the "types" of your well-being (physical, financial, social, mental, spiritual and emotional). By understanding these "broad and deep" perspectives of well-being, you will be better equipped to take on the craft of developing your well-being ultimatum strategic action plan and optimizing your well-being.

CHAPTER 3:

THE WHOLE WELL-BEING STORY: WHY SUBJECTIVE AND OBJECTIVE VIEWS MATTER IN THE OPTIMIZATION OF YOUR WELL-BEING

In chapter 1, we discussed why Super Heroes like you may need a well-being ultimatum. In chapter 2, we discussed how stress, crisis, compassion fatigue and burnout foster ill-being as opposed to well-being, and how they can impede your ability to handle the stresses that occur both in your work (your "calling" to heal, lead and/or serve others) and in your life. In this chapter, we will unpack the science of well-being -- to explore what well-being is and isn't, and what that means for you, your work/life balance, your longevity and your overall quality of life.

If you ask your friends what the term well-being means, you will no doubt hear many answers. If you ask a group of scholars representing a diverse array of fields in the humanities, natural sciences and the social sciences, you will also hear many answers. As one scholar I know mentioned to me when I explained that I would be studying well-being as part of my doctoral dissertation work -- "the only thing that well-being scholars agree on is that none of us can agree on what well-being is or isn't."

Taken from a scientific perspective, you have to admit this is actually a bit funny. If you are a chemistry scholar, you know what chemistry is. If you train to become a physician, you know what medicine is. And yet, in well-being science, the one thing that we well-being scholars agree on is that we don't know exactly what well-being is or isn't -- because it is largely defined and experienced by each individual in a different way.

But that ambiguity didn't stop me from trying to figure out what it was -- as a person and as a scholar. In fact, my entire professional life has been dedicated to either finding, promoting, coaching and/or researching well-being. Early in my career, I studied and created theatre in an effort to better understand life through the power of story-making and story-telling. Later, I studied biomechanics (kinesiology), yoga therapy and the Pilates method to understand the "mind/body connection" that many would say is a hallmark of living well, and achieving well-being. And most recently, I dedicated four years of my life (2010 - 2014) to studying well-being and its promotion as part of my doctoral work.

After all that time, energy, research, and contemplation, I can tell you that essentially I have come full circle. Well-being is unique to each of us, and largely depends on our stories -- the ways we tell them to ourselves, to our family and friends, and to the world.

I came to that conclusion though only after I tracked what other scholars had to say about it -- and not all of them would agree with me. I'll try to summarize the scholarship here, knowing that (1) no matter how succinct I try to be, it will still become complicated and (2) not all scholars will agree with my take on well-being that you're about to see. Still, if you are making a well-being ultimatum, you should at least have an understanding of the disagreements and the discourse surrounding well-being.

So here goes.

Your well-being comes in two essential types: subjective and objective well-being. Subjective well-being is where most well-being scholarship lies; this approach to well-being assumes that the individual gets to decide what well-being is, and how they rate their experience of this definition. This is why well-being is so hard to define from this perspective: each individual conceptualizes what it means to "live well" and/or in a "good life" in their own unique way based on their own unique circumstances and assumptions.

We find that subjective well-being (SWB) occurs in three main types (categories). First, some scholars believe that SWB is about how you feel about the experience of your life and/or your lived experiences; happiness is an example of this. You can be happy about the fact you had lunch today; and you can be happy you met the man of your dreams. Sometimes our happiness can get complicated when we try to apply it in to specific dimensions of our life; happiness in one area does not always imply happiness in another area.

The second type of subjective well-being that is widely-accepted is based on how you evaluate your life and/or your lived experience; life satisfaction is an example of this. You can be satisfied with the way your day went (because you were able to spend time with a friend) and/or you can be satisfied with the fact that your job is rewarding. Like happiness, sometimes your life satisfaction can get messy and complicated -- when you shrink and/or expand what it is you are evaluating (i.e. your life, your work, your work/life balance, etc.). For example, your recent promotion may have been something you were professionally "satisfied" but personally "dissatisfied" by. If your promotion disrupts the amount of quality time you have with your family and friends, you may find the promotion as not bringing you the work/life balance dimension of life satisfaction, even if it did bring you a sense of professional advancement (life) satisfaction.

The third type of subjective well-being can be a combination of these two "affect" (happiness) and "cognitive" (life satisfaction) SWB types; quality of life measures are an example of this. These hybrid instruments are most-often used to measure your comprehensive well-being. The well-being WHO-5 measure used in this book is an example of such a quantitative "hybrid" measure. Your quality of life can change easily over time, depending on life events and your perceptions (feelings and thoughts) about them.

So, if we stop here for a moment, you can see why so many people have difficulty in living well. The (affect) experiences of their well-being that result from the multiple dimensions of their life don't always get along; the (cognitive) evaluations of these experiences and their life as a whole don't always get along; and these experiences and their evaluations are not always internally consistent. Happiness does not always imply life satisfaction and vice versa. What makes us happy or satisfied in one part of our life may make us unhappy in other parts, and vice versa. Quality of life does not always stay consistent when we measure our experience of life over the course of a week, a day and/or a year.

Subjective well-being, according to most scholars, is therefore truly in the eye of the beholder: we get to decide if affect, cognition, and/or a combination of the two are important to us in the ways that we understand well-being, and we get to decide what life experiences will bring us closer to these self-designed and self-interpreted standards.

My colleague and friend Erik Angner uses the term "preference hedonism" (Angner, 2009) to describe this self-directed nature of subjective well-being. His work shows that when we are living in the ways that we prefer, we are more likely to be happy. But he also challenges all of us to consider these preferences against legal and moral structures; just because we are thinking, feeling and/or doing what we want does not mean that it is good for us, those around us and/or for society.

That next layer of complexity – where our own needs meet up with and/or against social, legal, ethical and moral structures -- is where the other half of well-being comes in (the objective half). Objective measures of well-being that exist can all be summarized as "other-based evaluations of your life and/or lived experiences". Your safety, your security, and your welfare can be self-evaluated (looked at subjectively by the individual) but these dimensions of well-being are actually best-understood when some "other" party evaluates them. An "other" can be a person, a group, an expert, and/or an agency.

For example, my sons may believe that their safety and security is high but they may not know that I perceive their choice to be out past curfew as a not-safe option (which jeopardizes their well-being). I, as their parent and in this case the "other," am considering factors that they may not have thought of or known about, such as crime rates, the increased prevalence of drunk drivers after 1 am, and the sleepiness that they may experience at the wheel if they drive after curfew. I see their being out late as inviting these adverse consequences, and therefore "bad" for their (objective) well-being. At the same time, they are experiencing the fun of being out with their friends (affect) and they are happy about the fact that they can do so (cognition) – so their subjective well-being rating is high.

We have a problem here in this case study and in most evaluations of well-being - subjective and objective well-being do not always get along.

Here's another example to indicate the dialectic tension that exists between one's subjective (self-rated) and objective (other-evaluated) well-being. I can be happy that I am drinking water (affect); feel satisfied with myself that I am maintaining my health by drinking water (cognition); and therefore perceive/rate my well-being as high for the day (subjective well-being). However, I may not know that someone who was ill used the glass without my knowing (I am unknowingly more susceptible to disease) and/or that the water I am drinking has a public health-concern (an unannounced health crisis). Subjectively, I understand the drinking of the water to be a good idea. An "other's" evaluation (my friend, my doctor, my public health official) would know otherwise, and would challenge my positive self-rating with a more negative (objective) appraisal.

Have I confused you yet? Rest assured, I was confused too - for two years as I chased these various components of well-being and tried to define it. In fact, the more I tried to define well-being, the more contradictions I seemed to find.

This realization that well-being definitions can be contradictory and also confusing, led me to offer the following alternative approach to "defining" well-being:

> Although well-being is difficult for scholars and the public to define, it functions as a communication (sensemaking) process in which the individual makes sense of health outcomes, role identities, life situations, and/or lived experience. (Carmack, 2014)

As you can see, this approach puts you in the driver seat: it implies that you get to make sense of your life as you need to and as you want to, and that as you make sense of your life, so too will your well-being improve. As mentioned above, I have come full circle to believe that it is the ways we tell ourselves our story, the ways we tell our stories to others, the ways that others receive that story, and the meanings that are created in the world from these acts of story-telling that collectively influence both our subjective (self-rated) and objective (well-being).

This is why this text recommends in the creation of your well-being ultimatum plan, that you combine both self-appraisals of your well-being with objective ones. In order to optimize well-being we have to see both of its sides: we need to be sure that the process of defining, assessing, evaluating, and strategizing our well-being acknowledges both our subjective and objective well-being perspectives. If we focus solely on objective well-being approaches (i.e. others' appraisals of our life), then our unique and individual voice (and perceptions of what is and is not important) will be lost. And if we focus solely on subjective well-being approaches (i.e. we make sense of our life however we deem appropriate), then our self-rating will not be "checked" by external (other-based) assessment.

You will therefore see in the well-being ultimatum strategic planning process (chapter 5) that you will be asked to not only complete a well-being questionnaire (which will help you to assess your subjective well-being) you will also be asked to choose several key individuals in your life to (objectively) evaluate your well-being. In this way, you can potentially give yourself a "360 view" of your well-being, by receiving inputs and feedback from the people that represent your both sides of well-being.

For example, you may rate your quality of life as generally high (8 on a 10 scale), but you may have mixed feedback from your "team of experts." Your spouse may agree that your well-being is good; but your child may perceive you as more stressed than "well". Your doctor may perceive you as delinquent on your maintenance appointments (i.e. you missed your mammogram) and your lawyer may be still waiting for you to complete your will paperwork. In this example, you have a high subjective well-being but a mixed objective well-being result. In this case, you would develop a well-being ultimatum plan that helps you to optimize the areas of your well-being that are currently working well, while tackling the areas that are insufficient and/or delinquent – on both subjective and objective sides of the well-being house.

I encourage you to take a moment now and to consider what well-being means to you -- based not only on the discussion thus far but also about your life and how you live it. How would you self-rate it? How would others self-rate it?

Interestingly, the most common response I have received to that first question -- "what does well-being mean to you" -- is silence. Every person I have talked to pauses before they answer, on average for 2 – 3 seconds. This initial hesitation to answer the question is an indication that most people have trouble articulating, or defining the term well-being. In this moment of silence, I can almost see the computer that is their mind running an analysis trying to consider what well-being does and does not mean for them. Once they do come up with an answer, there is more often than not hesitation in their pace and/or in their tone. It is like someone is asking them to give a book report on a book they haven't read; they aren't sure if their answer is "right" for them or for me.

In my doctoral research process (Carmack, 2014), I conducted 38 in-depth (hour-long) interviews with individuals varying in age and demographic profiles. I began each interview asking all of these participants to explain what well-being meant to them. Here is a breakdown of the key terms used responses. Keep in mind that each participant used an average of 3-4 responses, which is why there are almost 4 times as many responses as there was participants (n=38). Take a look at the list below, and see if you recognize any dimensions of well-being that you would agree or disagree to. And, consider whether or not there are any dimensions of well-being that are not included on this list.

Mental	n=23
Physical	n=21
Healthy	n=18
Goals/Accomplishments	n=15
Emotional	n=14
Calm and Content (No stress)	n=14
Spirit	n=9
Balance in Life	n=9
Happy	n=8
Social	n=7
Taking Care of Self	n= 7
Hope	n=3
Wellness	n=1

As you can see from the data set above, only half (18) of the participants in my study used the term health or healthy to describe what well-being meant to them; only 8 of them used the term happy; and only 1 of them used the term wellness. Although this is but one study, these findings challenge the traditional practice of using the terms health, wellness and well-being interchangeably, and the traditional practice of using the terms happiness and well-being interchangeably. Both the diversity and the quantity of these answers support my premise here -- that well-being is much more complicated than traditional notions of it being synonymous with the terms "healthy" or "wellness".

Another interesting finding is that none of the participants used the objective well-being term welfare, or the subjective well-being terms quality of life or life satisfaction in their description of what well-being means to them. This is significant since these terms are often used in the literature to describe well-being; in fact, metrics based on these terms are widely-used to evaluate well-being. This may be caused in part by the fact that most people do not wake up saying "I have a high quality of life today" or "I have high satisfaction with my life today" – despite the fact that a survey may indicate that this result is or is not the case. Nevertheless, the fact that people do not say these terms is an important factor that well-being scientists like me should consider further when designing and analyzing research studies -- are we really measuring quality of life, life satisfaction and/or welfare? Or is there something else we should be looking at?

One way to bring these theoretical questions into a real-world context, is through a case study. You will see the competing needs of my subjective and objective sides of well-being present themselves in very real ways.

CASE STUDY (ME)

I wake up knowing that I have a big project due for work by 10 am. I choose not to go on my morning run because I want to meet the deadline, and I do not perceive that I have the time to both run and complete the project. This decision came out of my desire to "optimize my well-being" – specifically my physical well-being via my financial well-being. (My ability to function in the world is dependent upon my finances, which is dependent upon my career; if I don't come through for work then my financial well-being will be jeopardized).

My subjective self-rating of this decision is high, because I believe that my financial and physical well-being should take precedence, because it is a weekday.

However, despite the fact I would self-rate this decision as a good one, I may not have a full, 360 degree view of my whole well-being story. For example, I may not realize that my choice not to run is actually detrimental to not only my financial well-being, but also my physical well-being. This is because my personal trainer, if given the opportunity, would objectively evaluate my well-being as low. He would do this because he knows what I do not -- that this choice not to run will have a negative effect on both my longevity and also on my ability to write and think clearly. If I did not know that research shows that movement and exercise can increase our cognitive capability, I would not realize that my choice not to run was actually not the right choice for my financial well-being. I wouldn't know that running would have actually improved my performance on the short-term task at hand. I wouldn't know that what I thought was a good financial (subjective) well-being decision was actually a poor one (in terms of both my subjective and objective well-being)

As you will see in the well-being ultimatum planning section of this book (in Chapter 5), I suggest that you optimize BOTH your subjective and objective well-being by ensuring that you allow yourself to have both subjective and objective appraisals of your well-being. In the case study noted above, I would never have perceived my choice not to run as bad for my financial well-being if I had not received the objective appraisal of the personal trainer. Many people similarly fail to realize that what they think is good for them (subjectively) is actually not (when seen from both subjective and objective perspectives).

The reason I am so adamant about this recommendation -- to balance your subjective well-being self-ratings with objective other-based evaluations -- is because this is the fundamental problem that Super Heroes have. Those who live to heal, lead, and/or serve others as healers are so concerned with helping others (living to their meaning and purpose, a dimension of subjective well-being) that they often forget to balance this drive with objective well-being practices. This is why the Well-Being Ultimatum plan included in this book will ask you to commit to your self-care on a daily basis, your social support on a weekly basis, and your use of services on a monthly basis.

All three of these "S's" (self-care, social support and services) will help you to build your inner and external capacities, and in so doing, to balance and optimize your subjective and objective well-being. Self-care will not only help you to boost your mood and/or your quality of life (both subjective well-being dimensions), it will also help you to manage and prolong your longevity (objective well-being). Social support will help you to also have a higher mood and quality of life, and will ensure that you have some "accountability" for your life choices by those who play important roles in your life. Services will likewise help you to ensure that your subjective and objective well-being needs are met; service-providers can not only help us to feel good in the moment (fix a problem for us) but can also help us to be cautious about areas that we may not have realized we had problems in in the first place. For example, we may feel good getting our current financial house in order (subjective well-being) but our financial planner may help us to also discover the importance of planning for our retirement now (objective well-being)

Because of the ability of these "three S's" to simultaneously optimize your subjective and objective well-being, I have built this entire well-being ultimatum plan around them. You will see in the planning section that I will ask you to commit to the following Self-Care practices on a DAILY basis: (1) movement and mobilization (don't think exercise exclusively although that counts); (2) practicing mindfulness and positive self-talk, especially gratitude, ideally to begin your day; (3) eating as "clean" as possible and as needed for your daily fueling and medical requirements; (4) detoxing yourself from electronics/digital devices for at least 1 hour per day, ideally at the end of your day; (5) attending to your daily medical needs as appropriate (i.e. taking medication for a chronic illness or attending a daily meeting for a recovering program); (6) committing your whole self (mind, body and heart) to engaging in one non-work-related endeavor; and (7) sleeping at least 6.5 hours per evening.

Please note that if this seems like a long list, that may indicate that you really need to make the Well-Being Ultimatum; these are not outlandish requests. Each of the above recommendations are in fact all basic evidence-based guidelines for healthy living today. If it helps to feel less daunting, some of these areas can be combined. For example, your daily practice of movement may also be combined with your mindfulness practices and your "whole self" commitment to a non-work endeavor.

Committing to the second "S" -- social support -- on a WEEKLY basis will ensure that you do not become isolated; this will help you to enjoy the "physiologic bump" we get when we spend time with those we love (subjective well-being). Ii will also decrease the likelihood that you will have a false sense of security in your life choices and endeavors (i.e. help you to manage your objective well-being). Our family and our dear friends have a way of calling us out when we make choices that we think are "a good thing" but may not actually be so good for us. For example: have you ever had a friend who believes they are in a great relationship, but you are worried it isn't so healthy? You have the gift of being able to see their relationship objectively, even though your friend cannot because they are living in the subjective experience.

A weekly commitment to social support is not only important

to keep our relationship and other life choices in check; it is also an indicator of your ability to find work/life balance and to live "well". Those who are engaging in addictive behaviors (both workaholics and those addicted to substances) often withdraw from their major relationships -- partly because they are so consumed with their addiction and partly because they do not want to "face" the people in their lives they know may call them out on their maladaptive behavior. This is one of the ways we actually define addiction -- when choices we are making are causing trouble for our major relationships.

To illustrate this in a real-world example: a few years ago, I would often cancel my lunch and coffee dates at the last minute because something came up. I started to notice a pattern that the something that came up was always work-related. Sadly, the situation escalated to the point where I stopped scheduling coffees and lunch dates at all; unless they were work related. It was only through additional outside support -- therapy -- that I was able to see how destructive this pattern was, and to face the fact that I was exhibiting "textbook" workaholic behavior patterns. At the time I was canceling the appointments, my subjective well-being was high; however, my friends and family would have rated my (objective) well-being as low or at least challenged. It wasn't until a friend pointed out to me that I was canceling a lot of our coffee dates, that I considered that this pattern may not be so healthy -- and I pursued help for it.

So this well-being ultimatum will recommend that you make time for social support weekly in order to optimize your subjective and objective well-being -- both to ensure you have the accountability that comes from your deep relationships and to ensure that you are spending your work/life time in ways that are adaptive (and not maladaptive). You get to decide how long these "bouts" with your friends and family members may be -- and what form they take (a workout, a Skype call, a lunch date). But you don't get to let this weekly commitment go; because your social support is a vital component to ensuring that your well-being needs are being kept in balance. The good news is that we really do know that social support is not only good for you (optimizing your well-being as discussed here). Social support makes us feel good; my dissertation work (Carmack, 2014) found that social support is not just correlated with -- it predicts -- all dimensions of well-being (physical, mental, emotional, social and comprehensive).

The third "S" that I recommend for your Well-being Ultimatum, in addition to self-care daily and social support weekly-- is "Services" on a MONTHLY basis. This "S" is a bit more complicated to explain than the first two, because how you enact this "S" really does depend upon the particular elements of your life and your life story. Your "service" dimension of your well-being ultimatum is admittedly a "first world problem"; it is something that is a unique challenge for those of us Super Heroes living in developed countries. It is an evolutionary trade we have made for our modern lifestyles. While those in less-developed countries may conceptualize their "service" component as the individual's willingness to seek out help and support from others on an informal basis, those living in more-developed countries will do this as an "act of commerce" (hiring and/or bartering with them).

No matter how we get these services (through donation, through bartering, and/or through hiring), we all will find ourselves from time to time having stresses (life events) for which we need external support (See chapter 2). Please keep in mind that under services I not only group the "services" that we need for our legal, financial and professional lives, I also include any service that enhances your physical, social, mental, spiritual and/or emotional well-being. These service needs can include -- but are not limited to -- your basic legal, financial, ethical, mental, physical, medical needs. They can also include other "first-world" needs such as your car's needs for ongoing maintenance and mechanical work and your personal "beauty-related needs".

Another reason why this particular "S" (service) is especially difficult to employ in your well-being contract, is because Super Heroes like you -- those who live lives dedicated to healing, leading and/or serving others – often have some pretty strong biases about which services they consider acceptable and those that are not.

For example, many Super Heroes that I have worked with have no problem asking for help with the updating of their hair and/or nails, the drawing up of their will, or the maintenance of their car. However, these same Super Heroes do not believe it would be appropriate to visit a mental health therapist and/or a physical therapist. They believe this because they (falsely) view these or other "service needs" (such as mental and/or physical difficulties) as something that they can just push through.

Super Heroes don't like admitting that they need these services, because it means that they are vulnerable. They (falsely) perceive that their request for service help indicates that their ability to heal is compromised in some way. To quote an old commercial from the 1980's – Super Heroes don't like to have you (or anyone) see them sweat. (For more on how your willingness to show, rather than hide, your vulnerabilities -- and how this is actually an expression of power -- please see the inspiring work of Brene Brown). Of course, what Super Heroes often fail to see is that if they would only just ask for help, their capacity to be of service would be strengthened (and not diminished). As noted in Chapter 2, they need backup.

Together, these three S's (self-care, social support and services) will help you to ensure that both your subjective and your well-being needs are not only met, but optimized. This Well-being Ultimatum is dependent upon your ability optimize both your subjective and objective well-being. And it is for good reason -- your subjective well-being (your "preference hedonism" to use the term from Dr. Angner, 2009) only tells one half of the your well-being story. Research shows that narcissists, addicts and workaholics all self-rate their well-being as high; the self-involved are happy even when that self-involvement is not good for them and/or is not good for others.

Your Subjective (Self-defined and self-interpreted) and Objective (Other-based) Well-Being Components Give Us Your Whole Well-Being Story

To summarize, this book – this guide to creating your Well-being Ultimatum -- is built on the following assumptions. First, the book begins with the assumption that your well-being is optimized when you assess, monitor and evaluate your well-being both subjectively (self-rate) and objectively (engage in other-based evaluation processes). Second, it assumes that your inner and external capacities can both be enhanced in order to optimize the subjective and objective dimensions of your well-being. Third, it challenges you to build these inner and external capacities by practicing the "three S's": committing to daily self-care, weekly social support, and monthly services as needed to handle the stresses that occur in your work and in your life. And fourth, it reminds you that these capacity-building, optimizing efforts are not only important for improving your quality of life and your longevity -- they will help to prevent the compassion fatigue and/or burnout that often plagues Super Heroes (Strategic Healers) like you.

It is my hope that you find this Well-being Ultimatum "3 S" framework to be a valuable tool. It is designed to help you to strategically optimize both the complexities of your well-being (how it is difficult to define, measure and evaluate because it is largely self-interpreted); and the contradictions of your well-being (how your subjective and objective dimensions of your well-being won't always get along).

To be clear, I really do want to help you and I I really do not wish to confuse you!

By recognizing these complexities and contradictions up front,

I hope to prepare you for succeeding in the process of making and managing your Well-being Ultimatum. I want you to know "what you are in for" so that you can better navigate and negotiate your way through these complexities, and contradictions in order to define, live and evaluate the life that really is ideal for you. You will therefore be less likely to suffer the ill-being effects that result from the tidal shifts of well-being that can occur on a day-to-day or even hourly basis.

As any leader will tell you – when you see a challenge coming, it is a lot easier to strategically address it. What at first seems like an overwhelming challenge can actually become an opportunity.

In the same way, I hope that sharing these complexities and contradictions of well-being will help you to strategically address them. And, I hope that encouraging you to get a full, subjective and objective view of your well-being will enable you to create your own kind of well-being opportunity – to really make a Well-being Ultimatum once and for all.

With this understanding of the importance of examining your well-being from both subjective and objective perspectives, in order to see and optimize your whole well-being story, the discussion next turns to the major players of that story – your dimensions (types) of well-being.

CHAPTER 4
KOSHA-BASED WELL-BEING COACHING: HOW TO GET YOUR (PHYSICAL, MENTAL, EMOTIONAL, SOCIAL, & SPIRITUAL) WELL-BEING DIMENSIONS TO ALL GET ALONG

You have probably heard a friend say at one point or another "I have a theory…". You may have even posited one or two yourself. I used to have a "theory" when my children were very young that they were only loud when I got onto the telephone. This is not a widely-known theory, but it was "my theory" nonetheless. When I talked to other Moms, they would often agree that this was a justified theory – many of them found it true for their lived experience as well. A scientist may not consider this a "legitimate" theory but it was true for me and my lived experience nonetheless.

There are a variety of theories and models that seek to explain dimensions of our life – some of which are more accepted than others, and some of which have been tested more than others. Anyone can come up with a theory. However, as far as science is concerned, only theories that have been legitimately tested in the scientific process are true "theories". As noted by Glanz (1997), a theory is:

> "A set of interrelated concepts, definitions, and propositions that presents a systematic view of events or situations by specifying relations among variables in order to explain and predict events or situations." (Glanz, 1997).

In my example earlier, I found my behavior of picking up the phone to be predictive of my children's making of loud noise. These events (variables) may or may not have been related, but to me there was definitely a relationship there. While this "theory" may have been true for me, it would need further (reliability and validity) study in my own life and testing in the lives of other Moms to determine if this was really a "theory" or just a phenomenon.

Somewhere between something being a phenomenon -- a series of coincidental events that catches our attention -- and a theory is a model. There are several types of models. A model can be a budding theory; preliminary testing reveals that the ideas in a prospective theory are valid but further testing is needed in order to be sure this is the case. A model can also sometimes be a very specific and/or new lens on a pre-established theory; a way to apply a theory into a particular situation or circumstance. Sometimes (although not always) the terms model and framework are considered synonymous; in this discussion I will use these terms interchangeably.

Why am I discussing theories, models and frameworks here? Because, in this chapter, I offer you several models for the optimization of your well-being.

Let's begin this discussion by examining traditional approaches to health and wellness coaching. Although many people may consider health, wellness and well-being to all be essentially the same thing, they aren't necessarily. For the sake of this discussion, I'm going to ask you to assume three things. First, consider health as your status -- whether you have disease or not. Second, consider wellness as how you are (or aren't) strategically managing this health status by engaging in behaviors that either prevent illness and/or manage it. And third, consider your well-being as your experience of the other two. (These are not the only definitions of these terms of course, but for the sake of this discussion we can start from here).

Most health and wellness coaches encourage their clients to consider their life more from these health outcome and/or wellness viewpoints, and not necessarily from a well-being perspective. This means that they usually focus on health and wellness behaviors and strategy, and either ignore or minimize the importance of one's lived experience (or well-being). This is not because they wish to ignore well-being; it is usually because they assume that the act of maintaining one's health and optimizing one's wellness will manifest (create) well-being. However, as we have seen throughout this book, there is a lot of tension between what is good for us (health and wellness behaviors) and our experience of the good life as we define it (our well-being).

The following diagram illustrates a typical wellness wheel, which is used in many health and wellness coaching programs as a way to assess, evaluate, and/or coach a client to achieve "balance" in their life and/or strategically optimize health and wellness outcomes.

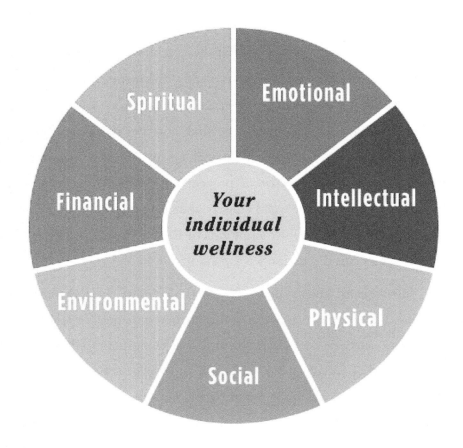

Source: University of Utah, Center for Student Wellness (2015)

When using the above wellness wheel (or others like it), most health or wellness coaches would ask you to look at each section of the pie chart, and to evaluate (self-rate) each area of your life in terms of how you perceive you are doing well, or not well. They might even ask you to color in each area relative to your performance; coloring in the parts that you deem successful and keeping blank the parts you feel overwhelmed or challenged by.

If your total wellness wheel ends up colored in a "lopsided" fashion (for example, your social piece is filled in because you feel good about your relationships but your financial piece is empty because you do not feel you have enough resources to function well) then the health or wellness coach would help you to shift your attention, priorities and behaviors in order to achieve balance within each piece, as well as across the (wellness) wheel of your life.

A more complex version of this wellness wheel, is found in the Total Force Fitness (TFF) framework, developed by the U.S. Department of Defense and utilized in the military health system. (See page 88 for a depiction of the TFF framework). This "wheel" is actually an octagon, and recognizes the importance of standard wellness components (physical, social, psychological) as well as often-missing components (such as behavioral, medical, and dental).

The Total Force Fitness (TFF) framework implies that the U.S. military's ability to be "fit" (and able to respond to security needs as appropriate) is directly dependent upon each service members ability to be "fit" in each of these areas. For example, units cannot deploy all of their personnel if individual soldiers or airmen fail their exams.

Both of these examples of wellness wheels (and there are many others out there in the world of health and fitness promotion) assume that the individual experiences the dimensions of their life separately, and that this experience is largely driven by behavior. What you are about to see – my Kosha approach to well-being – challenges the assumptions laden in these other wellness wheel approaches in three key ways.

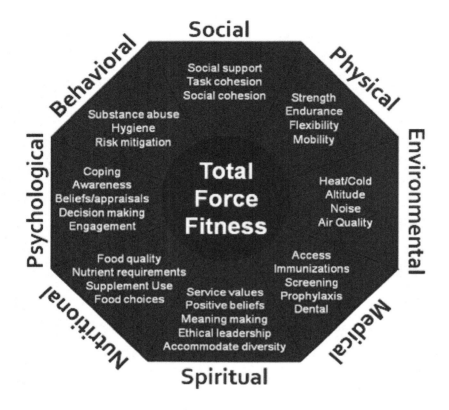

Source: Joans, et. al. (2010)

First, it assumes that our physical, social, mental, spiritual and emotional experiences of our life are not bound to our individual health outcomes and/or our wellness behaviors. This means that our well-being is not necessarily dependent upon how "sick" or "healthy" we are or how much we are or aren't engaged in "healthy" behaviors. Second, it assumes that financial well-being is a sub-component of our physical well-being, because the physical well-being layer refers to our ability to "function well" in the world. This ability to function is as much dependent upon our physiology (as discussed in chapter 2) as is our financial well-being.

Third, the model recognizes that life is a biopsychosocial experience. So, one way to evaluate our experience of life (our well-being) is to not tackle it by "cutting it up into separate pieces" as is done in most wellness wheel-based evaluations. Instead, the kosha approach asks you to view life from the vantage point of your mind, body, heart, spirit and life (relationshps). This means that the different aspects of your well-being (physical, social, mental, spiritual and emotional) each have their own identity and influence on your lived experience and well-being.

Fourth, this proposed Kosha model of well-being recognizes that your comprehensive well-being is dependent as much on the optimization of each dimension (type) of well-being, as it is to the recognition that all of these dimensions are interrelated. Each layer (dimension of your well-being) does not function separately (as is implied in other traditional wellness models); instead, there is an ongoing ripple effect between all of the layers. Optimization occurs for your well-being when each type of well-being is optimized, and when all of these types of well-being are also interacting in ways that support your subjective and objective well-being.

Your well-being ultimatum strategic planning process will therefore not require you to "cut up your life" into the pieces of your health and the dimensions of your well-being. It will not ask you to build your entire plan around your health outcomes - as is the case in most health and wellness coaching -- but will instead ask you to build your plan around your inner and outer experience of your life as it is.

I need to emphasize here, that this approach is not meant to ignore your health outcomes -- I want you to continue your medications, your therapy, and anything else a clinician has recommended for you. But I will be asking you to disassociate from that somewhat narrow (medical) approach to starting with what is wrong (illness) and to instead subjectively and objectively evaluate your lived experience (of which health and wellness are only part).

Simply put, instead of trying to get you to manage your health strategically by improving your health and wellness through behavioral shifts, and hoping that your well-being will improve as a result, I will take you through a reversed version of that process.

Analyzing the dimensions of your well-being will help you to see where you are realizing and losing power (where you are and aren't living strategically). This process will help you to redirect your assumptions, your behaviors and/or your perceptions accordingly in order to optimize your well-being. It is my hope that this process will not only improve your well-being, but also positively influence your health and wellness outcomes too.

As you may have noticed, I've been referring to my Kosha model of well-being as just that – a model. This is because it is from a social science perspective, it is a new (and untested) framework. However, from a yoga therapy and Ayurvedic science perspective, the idea is not so new. The Koshas have helped thousands of people for the past 5,000 years to understand their lives in ways that enhance their well-being (even if that was not what they were calling it at the time).

So, suffice it to say that I am calling this a "Kosha model of well-being" because I want to recognize that (1) this is a new (untested) model from a modern well-being science perspective and that (2) the model links the time-honored Koshas of Yoga to modern social science in a way that slightly "adjusts" the koshas with well-being details.

To my knowledge, this linking of the science of well-being studies to the Koshas is new and is limited to my own work in the field with clients, teams and organizations, and in my own life. In fact, it was very surprising to me when I reviewed the literature (conducted a scope of current scholarship) and discovered that the widely-accepted and 5000-year old system of the Koshas has not yet been applied or linked to the science and/or promotion of well-being (at least not in the formal literature)

No matter what you may call them (a phenomenon, a model, a framework, a theory or something else), the Koshas serve as a powerful and easy-to-understand methodology (model) for appreciating the multiple dimensions (faces) of your well-being. In Chapter 3, I explained that we need two viewpoints to truly optimize your well-being: the integration of both self-based (subjective) and other-based (objective) perceptions, evaluations, and monitoring is a fundamental requirement for your ability to have a 360 degree, holistic perspective on whether or not you are living well. In this chapter, we will unpack the specific dimensions of your well-being, namely your physical (body), mental (mind), emotional (heart), social

A Kosha / Well-being Model

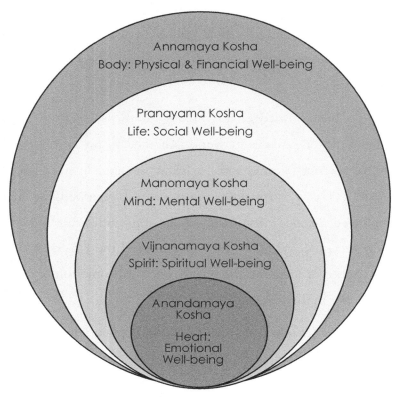

Annamaya Kosha
Body: Physical & Financial Well-being

Pranayama Kosha
Life: Social Well-being

Manomaya Kosha
Mind: Mental Well-being

Vijnanamaya Kosha
Spirit: Spiritual Well-being

Anandamaya
Kosha

Heart:
Emotional
Well-being

Purushamaya Kosha
"Pure consciousness"
(Deeper Than + Beyond Sheath Form)

(life/relationships) and spiritual (sense of meaning and purpose/faith/hope). Each of these faces of well-being can and should be examined both subjectively and objectively; their collective whole (comprehensive well-being) can also be examined subjectively and objectively.

Conveniently, the Kosha model of well-being can help to

summarize the dimensions (faces) of your well-being quite well. The term "Kosha" is the word that yoga philosophers and practitioners have used for many centuries to describe the "layers" around your soul. In fact, the word Kosha means "sheath" or "layer" in Sanskrit. Devout yoga masters will tell you that each layer (or Kosha) symbolizes a different layer (aspect) of your human experience.

The diagram of the Kosha/Well-being model illustrated in this chapter indicates how the koshas are conceptualized; they are a series of concentric circles similar to a target board or an onion. They have also been referred to having a similar expression as "Russian nesting dolls" – to indicate deeper and deeper layers of our lived experience. As you will see in the description of each layer (Kosha) to follow, the Koshas imply that beneath our "physical" experience of our life, we experience different layers (dimensions) related to our breath; mind; spirit; and emotions.

Annamaya Kosha

Sanskrit Translation:	"Food Sheath"
Well-Being Dimension:	Physical Well-being; Financial Well-being
"Body"	Our lived experiences (doing) in the world
Well-Being Measures:	Health Behavior and/or Medical Questionnaires (logs; screenings); Functional Health Assessment; Comprehensive Well-Being (WHO-5); Emotional Vitality; Financial Well-being

The translation from the Sanskrit term "Annamaya" is "food sheath" but this sheath refers to all of the needs and functions of your physical body (not just your ability to metabolize food). In my well-being approach to the Koshas, I consider this Annamaya kosha to be connected to your ability to function daily -- your ability to do what it is you have to do and what you want to do.

I place financial well-being in this layer, as a sub-component to physical well-being, because financial well-being influences the ways that we live and function in the physical world. Without financial resources, we can't buy food that is fuel; we can't ensure our personal security and welfare; we can't engage in activities that we need to accomplish and those that we want to accomplish; and we can't support the people that we care about. Our physical well-being (Annamaya kosha) depends on both physical, and financial functionality or well-being.

Please note that this layer is NOT about infirmity, illness, or disability; it is about function, access and quality of life. For example, someone who is wheel-chair bound may have a high sense of physical well-being, if they are able to accomplish the daily tasks that they choose to do and those that they want to do. Their 'disability' does not have to mean an adverse effect on their function. Conversely, someone who has no "physical ailments" may have poor physical and/or financial well-being if they are unable to function in their life in the way that they want to.

Pranayama Kosha

Translation:	"Life force extension"
Well-Being Dimension:	Social Well-being
"Life"	Relating in our relationships, communities

Well-Being Measures: Interpersonal Communication Competence; Social Support; Compassion Fatigue Questionnaire; Burnout Questionnaire

This sheath represents your overall "energy level" and your energy balance. In Sanskrit, the word "prana" refers to both your breath, and your overall "life force." The word "yama" means restraint; but in the term "pranayama" the term "ayama" is used which means to "extend or to draw out".

Not surprisingly, I have "matched" social well-being to the Kosha Pranayama second layer, because the ways that we function in our social relationships is directly correlated with our energy level. If we allow others to "walk all over us", we have too much in-flow and we have no power in our relationships. Conversely, if we have all outflow and we walk all over others, we can become over-bearing, narcissist, and definitely ineffectual as healers/ Serviceworkers/leaders.

Just as you can breathe all day without thinking about it, or you can make very specific efforts to extend, focus, direct and/or guide your breath for very specific results-- our overall sense of "life force" (energy and vitality) can also be something we don't think about at all, or it can be something that we very specifically extend, focus, direct and/or guide.

It is this Kosha that is especially susceptible to Compassion Fatigue and Burnout (discussed in chapter 2) because this is where your overall sense of "outflow and inflow" either achieve, or don't achieve balance. It is also where the balance between your inner and external capacities is indicated.

Compassion Fatigue can be conceptualized as a condition in which the Super Hero's outer sheath (Annamaya) becomes fragmented and/or withered; it therefore fails to protect this second, Pranayama sheath. The Super Hero's sense of "life force" is drained because they are all outflow, with no protective and/or supportive and/or receptive inflow. People who give out of love, but don't have the "boundary protection" of the outer-most protective (Annamaya) layer feel a ripple effect of imbalance that shows up in their Pranayama sheath. The Super Hero suffering from Compassion Fatigue may have a strong identify with their interior layers (of mind, heart, spirit) but the energy imbalance of their Pranayama layer and the fragmented Annamaya layers create a drain that is experienced both in their "life force" reality and in their "functional life reality".

From a Kosha perspective, Burnout is also a malfunction of these two layers, but is caused from an endurance (rather than imbalance) problem. The Super Hero hits an endurance wall because they are trying to "muscle through" their difficulties from a largely physical and/or financial perspective. They are trying to Make. Things. Happen. And are not allowing the flow of their deeper interior worlds (mind, spirit, and heart) to support their efforts. This is why they end of feeling detached, and may say statements like "my heart's just not in it anymore" – their physical, financial, and social realities (well-beings) are not in congruence with their mental, spiritual, and emotional ones.

If Compassion Fatigue is an over-identification with one's interior layers with a failure to recognize that receiving energy is importance to balance outflow; Burnout is an overidentification with one's exterior layers with a failure to connect with what is true in their heart, spirit and/or mind. In both cases, they are problems associated with our Social Well-being.

Finding balance in this layer is all about finding congruence between our inner and outer realities. Recognize the balance needed between your outflow to the world (your call to heal, serve and lead others) and your inflow (the personal, healing benefits you receive from acts of self-care, social support and/or service). By maintaining a cross-flow between these inner-outer and outer-inner relationships, you will be more likely to bolster your overall "life force".

One way that I personally find balance now in this layer – that was not always the case – is that I try to find time alone before I present information as a teacher or work with individuals as a healer. Just as I knew when I was a performer, I needed to spend time alone reviewing my lines and putting on my stage makeup before I went onstage, I know that I need to take time to be with myself before I go into these very outflow-based endeavors. Sometimes I meditate, sometimes I go for a walk, sometimes I practice yoga; these are all examples of self-care that gives me a sense of inflow that prepares me for all of the outflow I am about to take on. I also combine these self-care practices with other "services"; I have a funny superstition that I cannot deliver a good workshop if my nails are not done. I know this is a somewhat conceited worldview, but it works for me. I enjoy allowing the service provider (the nail technician) to share her gift with me, before I go share my gifts with others.

Manomaya Kosha

Translation: "Mind Sheath"
Well-Being Dimension: Mental Well-being
"Mind"   Perceptions of life, relationships, and world
Well-Being Measures: Life Satisfaction; Qual. of Life; Mindfulness

The term "Manomaya" is translated to "mind sheath", even though it is referring to both what we perceive and evaluate in our life (thoughts/mind) and how we experience those perceptions (through our senses). In this Kosha model of well-being, I refer to this as the layer of our mental well-being. It is directly related both to our mental health, and the interactive effect of the feeling (happiness) and thinking (life satisfaction) dimensions of our overall quality of life.

This layer helps to explain that our feelings become thoughts; and our thoughts become feelings; in fact, it is often hard to tell which comes first. It also helps to explain why our feelings and thoughts are not only felt in our mind and our hearts, but also how these influence our social well-being (Pranayama layer), our physical well-being and our financial well-being (Annamaya layer).

In this Kosha model of well-being, we buy into the idea that our thoughts and feelings have ripple effects into our relationships and into our bodies. It helps to explain the psychosomatic experiences of our lives – both in pain and in joy. It is also a fundamental assumption that yoga therapists like me make when we are working with people in movement; the experience of asking our client to move and to breathe is not just about optimizing these layers, it is about trying to get underneath these layers to the heart of the heart/mind.

Just like the five senses can only function if we are engaged in the real world (we can't smell, hear, taste, or see something if we are not aware of our external surroundings), this layer is not optimized unless we are tuned in. I can experience the air around me all day long; it is only when I tune into my sensory perception of my skin's sense of touch that I truly appreciate the experience of the air on my skin. The Manoymaya layer therefore asks us to check in with our deeper mental and experiential perceptions of our world; to be mindful of our thoughts and to find balance between the truth we see in the world, and the truth we are connected to in the deeper layers within.

Vijnanamaya Kosha

Translation: "Knowledge Sheath" or "Wisdom Sheath"
Well-Being Dimension: Spiritual Well-being
"Spirit"   Purpose: Call to serve, heal, and/or lead;
Well-Being Measures: Meaning and Purpose Questionnaire;
                         Engagement

From a traditional Kosha perspective, this layer refers to our spirit. I have found in my work with clients that this term – spirit – is loaded with meanings. Spirit can refer to the "esprit de corps" of our team. It can refer to the Holy Spirit as a mystical expression of God's power. It can refer to our sense of mood – our 'spirits' can be referred to as high or low to indicate how our day is going. And Spirit can of course refer to Source itself.

Just like the term Spirit is defined in many ways, Spiritual Well-being is also defined in many ways. For the sake of this Kosha model, we will assume that Spiritual Well-being refers to your having a deeper sense of meaning and purpose for your life. Notice I said a "deeper sense"; this is in keeping with the Kosha model, in which this spiritual layer is deep, underneath our mind (Manomaya) sheath, which is under our life force (Pranayama) sheath, which is under our and physical function (Annamaya) sheath.

As a Super Hero, you have a very deep and direct connection to this layer. That is both your strength – your Super Power – and the source of your imbalance (if you do not balance this strong layer with strength-laden efforts to the surrounding layers).

For those with strong spiritual and/or religious beliefs, this is also a layer in which our "call to service" that is beyond us, shows up for us. It is our connection to a higher voice -- of your higher, self-actualized Self (Maslow) and/or your Holy Spirit (Christianity). Although it is referred to as your "Higher" voice, it actually feels as though it is deep within us. We are the only ones who can "hear it". It is held deep within us; behind our mental perceptions, our relationships, and day-day (functional lives).

Visionaries – including Super Heroes -- usually have a very strong Vijnanamaya Kosha. As medical intuitive Carolyn Myss has stated in several workshops, "My interior sense of reality is now more real to me than what I see in the world". This Kosha helps to explain why visionary leaders are known for having strong "intuitions" about what is and isn't right for their company. You might say that they are directly tapped into awareness of this deep, intuitive wisdom layer.

However, the best healers, leaders, service members, are not only tapped into this layer, they are willing to listen to what lessons it offers them AND they balance those perceptions with their outer layer perceptions and experiences. Visionaries who don't take their great ideas out of this layer, and into the next layer out (thinking and feeling it through), and the next (getting it social support) and the next (getting it to manifest through physical and financial effort) fall short of having their ideas succeed. They literally get "stuck" without the benefit of these (layer) perspectives.

This is also one reason why visionaries and leaders don't always possess the same traits. You might say that leaders live more in their Pranayama and Annamaya (outer) layers and visionaries live more in their Vijnanamaya and Manomaya (inner) layers. The best and most visionary leaders find the ability to get all of these layers to get along – to negotiate an outcome that all inner and outer layers can agree on and deem successful.

As noted previously throughout this book, I recommend that you Super Hero make the time for the "3 S's" – self-care, social support, and services. Another reason this recommendation is made can be understood from the Kosha perspective. By engaging in these "3 S" behaviors, you will strengthen each of the layers that surround this layer – where your call to service lives. Self-care will strengthen your Annamaya layer; Social support will strengthen your Pranayama layer; and the use of services as needed for your ability to manage your life will strengthen your Manomaya layer. It's a three-part approach to protecting your Super Hero call to service.

Anandamaya Kosha

Translation: "Bliss Sheath" or "Joy Sheath"
Well-Being Dimension: Emotional Well-being
"Heart"   Experience of joy, peace, bliss, happiness
Well-Being Measures: Happiness; Self-Regulation; Self-Talk

When my children were very young, they had a song they would sing in preschool: "I've got the Joy, Joy, Joy, Joy, down in my heart." The Anandamaya Kosha is that joy.

As the innermost sheath, Anandamaya Kosha is your "happiness" sheath -- your bliss sheath. It represents your limitless capacity for joy, love, peace and happiness. Just like all good stories have a "happy ending" this sheath reminds us all that underneath our lived experience in the world (physical layer), our interaction with the world (life force layer), our perceptions of the world (mental layer), our call to serve the world (spiritual layer), lies our joy in the world (emotional layer).

In my work with clients, this worldview – that ultimately we are just happiness -- has provided some of the most profound shifts of well-being I have ever seen. This is because many of my clients (especially Super Heroes) come to me believing if they would just "do, think, and/or be" differently then their happiness will return to them. In other words, they are coming to see me because they want me to give them the "prescription" of what they should do, think, and or be differently in order to get to happiness.

The Kosha model (and this adaptation of it for well-being science) flips those assumptions on their head. It says that we all have unlimited joy. Our challenges in our experience in the world occur when we forget this – when we get so caught up thinking, doing, and/or trying to be something that we aren't. When any and/or all of our outer sheaths are out of balance, our joy is obstructed, or blocked.

While most of the time this idea – that joy really is deeply found inside of our hearts – is relieving, I do sometimes have clients who find this idea uncomfortable or even disturbing. Although not always, this is the case of an individual who has forgotten what joy feels like or who has been so traumatized by a physical, life, social, mental or spiritual event that they are completely blocked in their outer sheaths.

In these cases, I don't try to convince them that the model works for everyone – because it doesn't. (No model works for everyone). I also don't fault them for their reaction; in fact, I encourage them to be skeptical and to be in whatever reaction they may have. But I do ask them to at least open up to the idea that hope can live for them—whether it is through this model or through another. I ask them to invite hope to visit them, much like an old friend they haven't seen for a while. It doesn't always end up with their accepting the Kosha model – and that isn't the point. But it does give them a sense of hope that there will be a day where they can welcome their well-being again – wherever they find it. And as the work of Seligman has found, hope is a key foundation of our well-being.

Purushamaya Kosha

Translation: "Pure consciousness"

You may have noticed in this Kosha model of well-being, this sheath does not have a type of well-being attached to it, and it is does not refer to a specific dimension of our life: (body, life, mind, heart, spirit). It doesn't get a "ring" on the diagram either. This is because it is indicative of our connection to a greater consciousness that is beyond our ability to comprehend and/or give a name. It is beyond the limitations of a new circle, any of the other circles. It is beyond definition; it can't be bound by a circle on a chart no more than we can bind consciousness. It just Is.

It is therefore not surprising that many descriptions of the Koshas do not even recognize this as a sheath -- it is more of an assumption that when all of our Koshas are aligned, we will tap into this "pure consciousness". For those who are religious and/or spiritual, this layer can be considered God, Spirit, the Light, Source, and/or Brahman him/her/itself. However, for those who do not have these world/spirit/religious views, it can have a different meaning all together; that is entirely the point.

In totality, this Kosha model (approach) to well-being enables us to find one way to help explain the different dimensions of our well-being, and how each of these dimensions influences its fellow dimensions. It helps to explain how your well-being can be experienced physically, socially, mentally, spiritually, and emotionally; and, it helps to explain how any life event is experienced in all of these multiple (well-being) ways.

You might imagine that each life event (stressor) sends a "shock wave" through all of your koshas; each layer experiences and/or adapts to the stressor in its own unique way, and flow between the koshas is as important as each individual kosha is itself. Sometimes a stressor (a surprise) gets "stuck" in a layer; we can't shake our physical exhaustion; or our ruminating thoughts. In these cases it is important that we seek (service and/or social support) help.

As noted by Dossey (1982), "Nothing happens in the Universe or in the physical world (including the physical body health) that does not have its correspondent on all planes of manifestation." It is vital that we recognize that the sum total of all of the Koshas, as well as the interactive flow between them, is as important as each unique dimension. Much like the biopsychosocial health model (Engel and Romano, 1977) the sum is greater than the parts and all parts relate to and contribute to the sum of our well-being

So, the Kosha model approach to well-being science provides you with a powerful tool to acknowledge the interactive effect between the various components of your well-being. We can see through the Koshas that each unique dimension (layer) of your well-being has a story to tell, and all of these layers together tell an over-arching story about your comprehensive well-being. As noted previously, we can evaluate each layer, as well as their composite whole (Gestault) subjectively and objectively.

On a very practical level, the Koshas offer us a way to approach your Well-being Ultimatum. As you will see in the next chapter, we will create a well-being strategic action plan for each Kosha AND we will ensure that all of these layers (dimensions) of your well-being get along on a daily, weekly and annual basis. To me, this is the secret to work/life balance, longevity and quality of life -- that it isn't so much a matter of each of us balancing our work, life and play behaviors, as it is an act of negotiation between the competing demands of the various layers of our lived experience of well-being.

Using the Koshas as the key framework (model) for your well-being ultimatum is in keeping with the ways that the Koshas have been helpful to yoga practitioners for many years. As noted by, Radiant Life Yoga (2015):

> "The koshas comprise a practical and profound contemplative tool to help deepen our understanding of all aspects of ourselves…They help us to understand ourselves and others as multi-dimensional beings who need to come back into harmony with the soul in order to achieve health." (Radiant Light Yoga Website, 2015)

To recap, the Kosha model of well-being recognizes how your

functionality in this life (which includes both your physical and financial functionality); your life force (which is dependent upon your relationships and the balance between your in-flow and outflow); your perceptions (which is based on the mental experience of your thoughts, your feelings and your perceptions); your spirit (your sense of meaning and purpose) and your joy (your deep inner experience of blissful Truth) all influence your well-being. Each of these layers that surround your soul influences the other layers; together they also have a collective interactive well-being effect. An event for one layer (one dimension of your well-being), becomes an event for all. To dance, for example, is not just a physical experience. We may think of dancing as a physical act, but it becomes an event for our life/breath, our heart/emotions, our mind/thoughts, and our spirit/deep sense of self, as well as an expression of joy.

In order for you to better understand the value that the Koshas can have as a framework for making your Well-being Ultimatum, I would like to now lead you through an exercise which will help you to heighten your experience of them. You should know before we begin, that this (my) explanation of the Koshas. It is grounded both in the ways that they were introduced to me in the practice of yoga (philosophy and mind/body medicine), and to my own personal interpretations of how I experience them. This does not mean that this particular explanation matches with your own understandings of the Koshas, and it does not mean that you should limit yourself to my approach ("take") on the Koshas either. It is simply one (my) perspective to help to introduce you to the Koshas and/or to review them and their relevance to your well-being.

A Voyage Through Your Koshas - A Mindfulness Practice

[For an audio version of this exercise, please see my website, www.drsuziecarmack.com]

Find a comfortable position in a safe place, and close your eyes. Notice your breath, and allow yourself to enjoy the gentle ebb and flow of your inhale and your exhale.

Now imagine that your Highest Self, or your Soul -- however you conceptualize it -- is standing in space. Think of this as the part of you that knows there's a you to know. You notice that there is space all around you. You are alone, but you do not feel lonely. You are peaceful. You are calm.

Surrounding your Soul is the experience and emanation of joy. Together your Soul and Joy circulate (dance!) until you feel a type of condensation. Like two gaseous substances that can become condensed into a liquid or a solid, your joy and your soul have condensed into something else. But it isn't heavy; its a very real feeling of bliss, that is deep within you. Feel this joy deep inside your heart, your bones, your mind. This is your happiness layer, or your Anandamaya sheath / Kosha.

Stay in this layer for as long as you need to and/or want to. Notice how it is beyond thoughts or actions. It is a pure and intoxicating feeling that feels light and free, and flows easily around you, through you and from you.

Surrounding this experience of your next breath is your ability to discern how you get to this feeling of joy, and how you share it -- the Vijnanamaya Kosha. Your spiritual well-being lives here, because you know that your well-being is strengthened when you make a difference in the lives of others -- helping them, leading them, or serving them. Your unique abilities to heal, lead, and serve others are in this layer, and the feeling that you have been called to take on these actions lives here too. Much like Superman must "break through" his clothing to get deep into his Super Hero role, the part of you that really is a Super Hero lives here, deep within you.

Here, there is a quiet yet strong sense of knowing what is and what is not right for you. Here, you really know yourself and you have the ability to truly perceive others -- without judgment. Super Heroes don't judge the people that they save; but they do see the many parts of the world that need saving. You can see here – very clearly.

Your sense of meaning and purpose is here too, as well as your sense of engagement. You experience "power" when your inner joy (Anandamaya kosha - where we just were); your ability to discern and know what is right for you (Vijnanamaya kosha - where we are now) and your perceptions of your life choices (Manyomaya kosha - the next layer out that you can see from here) are all in synchronicity with each other. As you breathe into this layer, notice the peace that comes from trusting your intuition and what you see beyond what the world sees.

Surrounding this experience is the next layer - Manyomaya Kohsa, or mind sheath. Here you have the ability to examine your lived experiences in your relationships, your community, and the role/s you play in the world. Your inner knowing and wisdom (Vijnanamaya kosha - where we just were) pushes into this layer in helping you get into the real world of your lived experience. The meanings you create surrounding what the world sees, and what you inwardly perceive occur here.

Here you feel a sense of calm and trust when your deeper layers (of bliss and knowledge) are in synchronicity with the meanings you are experiencing in your life choices and your relationships. You also feel out of work/life balance, out of sync, and/or out of touch when these inner and outer realities are not aligned well, or at least when they do not seem to be getting along.

Here you know whether you are satisfied, or not with your life, and if your life has an overall sense of quality (or not). You realize that this sense of life quality and life satisfaction isn't so much about the particular choices you are or are not making, but is about the congruence you have between your heart (Anandamaya kosha), your spirit (Vijnanamaya kosha), and your mind (Manomaya kosha).

Take a moment to breathe in this deep perception of your life - - in your heart, your spirit and your mind. Notice how all three of these layers are referred to as "deep koshas" but they are all somewhat "aerial views" of your life. They each ask you to perceive your lived experience in ways that are above (behind) our normal, everyday actions and consciousness – to get to the deeper meanings of our lives. Here, we have a deep appreciation for being alive, for the people who are in our lives, and a deep sense of knowing what is and isn't right for us. Our "core" values live here - beneath what the world can see.

Next, much like a seed suddenly takes shape and breaks through the earth to show itself as an evolving flower, the seeds of your core perceptions start to permeate into your relationships and your life. Here you bring your deep, internal experience of your well-being out into the open.

Here, in this Pranayama layer of well-being, we experience the transition from your inner world (of heart, spirit, and mind) with the interactions that you have in your life (outer world). With each breath you take, you trade between the inner world and outer worlds. In this layer, you do your best to keep the exchange between these worlds as even, as fully expressed, and as energizing as a very deep breath.

This Pranayama kosha invites you to see how you are influencing the world, and how that is kept in balance by how you are, or aren't allowing the world to influence you. If you feel that you are out of balance here, play with your breath-- a symbol of your prana or life force. If you need energy from the world, breathe a sense of vitality in with a deep and long inhale. To heighten the effect, breathe in longer than your exhale for several cycles, until you are no longer comfortable doing so. Conversely, if you need to release unused, stale and/or angry energy from your inner world, breathe out longer than you breathe in with a sense of clearing release. Remember your exhales are there to calm you, and your inhales are there to restore you.

It is here, in this layer, that we can understand not only the effects of our breath on our physiological systems, we can understand how our inner and external capacities must be kept in balance. We realize that our well-being is dependent upon inner congruence -- between our heart, spirit and mind -- and on keeping these deeper aspects of our well-being congruent with our (outer layer) experiences of and interactions with the world. This experience of the world happens with every breath we take, and in every choice that we make.

Pause here to perceive your overall sense of flow -- how your inner capacity (of heart, spirit and mind) is or is not in balance with your external experience of the world. Are you expending more energy in restoring the world (i.e. being a Super Hero) without restoring yourself within? Or are you trying to balance your external drive to help, heal, lead and/or inspire others with your internal needs to restore your heart, spirit and mind? These questions will help you to discover whether your sense of (work/life) balance is compromised, and may help to explain your experience of compassion fatigue and/or burnout (if you find that you have it).

If you find yourself out of balance in this sheath, allow your self to welcome a downward, receiving, even absorbing energy. Much like a plant needs fertilizer, water, and love to survive and thrive, you do too. Like sunshine warms our skin, allow the warmth of the feelings of love and compassion to be absorbed through your skin and bones (symbols of your outer physical Annamaya layer) and into your deeper layers. Allow it to restore your breath, your mind, your sense of deeper purpose, and your joy.

Surrounding this experience of your energy balance and overall vitality (pranayama kosha), is your physical experience of the world. This is the plane in which others see you living this life -- your 'doing' of your lived experience. This Anandamaya kosha allows you to experience your time on this earth as a human -- your physiology lives here. You get to eat, to move, to digest, to sing, to dance, to sweat, to make love and many more physiological functions occur because of this sheath. Here you do your life.

You may notice that you feel physical well-being here if you are able to do the things that you want to do, and that your physical well-being may feel low if that is not the case. If this layer is compromised in any way, allow yourself to examine where this lack of peace is coming from. First, go within. Feel how your heart/joy, your spirit/sense of purpose, your mind/perception of your reality, and your life/relationships all influence your physical experience of well-being. Notice if any of these layers are "pulling" energy out of your physical well-being by taking too much of your physical energy and/or attention.

Now, notice how you can transform any and/or all of these layers to enhance your physical well-being. For example, notice how your breath can help you to feel better, even when experiencing physical discomfort. Notice how your decision to let go of anger with your colleague (life layer) makes you feel physically relieved. Notice how your satisfaction with your life and the quality of life is based in large part on your perceptions of what should and should not be occurring to you; and how you have the ability to change these perceptions (and manage stress) simply by changing these perceptions.

Notice how your call to heal, lead and/or serve others asks a lot of your physical well-being. Give yourself permission to be a human. Give yourself permission to be tired or energized or whatever physical experience you are having. Enjoy your human physiology – and the many different physical experiences it gives us.

Notice how your heart layer influences your physical well-being -- when you are happy deep within, you feel physically lighter. Allow yourself to free any fears, worries, doubts, angers, sadness from your heart -- which are all not found in the present moment -- as a way to free your physical experience of well-being. Notice how letting go of your negative feelings in any layer give you a new sense of peace, strength and vitality that you can really feel physically.

Finally, take a moment to allow your experience to evolve past these six layers and koshas, and to notice the flow between them and around them.

Allow yourself time to notice any blocks within each layer or between the layers. Allow something greater than you (consciousness) to free these blocks or at least hold them for you in an act of Grace. Notice how you feel charged internally and externally. Notice anything else that you feel.

This is yoga -- when body, mind, heart, life and spirit are experienced as one. Internally, you experience equanimity -- you feel peaceful, vital, and happy. This is enlightenment. Externally you know you have the ability and willingness to decide what is best for all of these dimensions of you, without reservation or hesitation. This is empowerment.

The space where your empowerment and enlightenment meet is equanimity. Here, your koshas (your body, mind, heart, life and spirit) are all in alignment internally and externally. In this rare space, you are one with yourself, with others, and the world. Your well-being is optimized here.

Take a deep breath, and open your eyes.

Although it is beautiful when these moments of equanimity are experienced, our life is usually a lot more complex. Usually, a life situation (stress) brings forth a more complicated array of reactions from our body, life, heart, mind and/or spirit, sending a ripple effect through our koshas (dimensions of well-being). Not only is each Kosha effected, there can often be a competing sense of reactions from each kosha.

When the needs of each Kosha is in conflict – this can be conceptualized as a kosha misalignment. This misalignment causes a well-being drain. When your ability to homeostatically balance your physical, mental, emotional, social and spiritual needs is compromised, your enlightenment and/or empowerment are compromised, and you find yourself out of work/life balance. In this misalignment, equanimity disappears, and ill-being occurs.

When you make your Well-being Ultimatum, you are therefore encouraged to remember the needs of each of your Koshas (well-being dimensions) and to ensure that they all "get along" (negotiate) with each other. As noted in chapter 1, your Superhero call to service (spiritual well-being kosha) can often times be at direct odds with your physical well-being kosha. You may forgo sleep, adequate nutrition, self-care practices and/or social support (dimensions of your physical and social well-being koshas) in order to meet the demands of your spiritual well-being. This lack of balance not only threatens your equanimity, it causes an energy drain that results in either compassion fatigue and/or burnout.

You can hopefully now see why I advocate for you to take on the "three S" framework for your Well-being Ultimatum, namely: your needs for self-care, social support and services. Your self-care practices will ensure that you are optimizing your maintenance (daily) well-being needs; your social support practices will ensure that you are balancing your inner (heart, spirit, mind) well-being needs with your outer (social, physical) well-being needs; and your services practices will ensure that you are monitoring, evaluating and addressing any deficiencies in any and/or all of your Koshas on a monthly basis. The 3 S's are your Kosha management system; they will help you to prevent and/or manage blocks to your physical, social, mental, spiritual, and/or emotional well-being, so that you can experience enlightenment, empowerment, and equanimity and therefore optimize your well-being.

CHAPTER 5
WELL-BEING ULTIMATUM:
HOW TO STRATEGICALLY DESIGN A WELL-BEING PLAN
AND CONTRACT THAT YOU CAN LIVE WELL WITH

If you have opened this book, and turned immediately to this chapter, I don't blame you. You know based on the title of the chapter, that this is "game day" – where we begin the real process of putting your Well-being Ultimatum plan together.

That said, I encourage you to become familiar with the four previous chapters first. I know you are busy, and you have a lot to do; you are a Super Hero after all. But, I assure you that your time in the proceeding chapters will be worth it. They will help you to understand who this Well-being Ultimatum is especially designed for (chapter 1); what benefits the well-being ultimatum planning and implementation process offers (chapter 2); what perspectives you should keep in mind when designing and evaluating your well-being (chapter 3); and how to better understand the ways that your dimensions of well-being live in both this planning process and in your life (chapter 4).

If I'm wrong, and you have already gone through these chapters, congratulations. It's time to get started.

WBU PLANNING PROCESS - BACKGROUND

If you are familiar with strategic planning processes, you know that they can be very complicated, or they can be surprisingly simple. They can be conducted very quickly, or they can take years to complete. They can be a very useful exercise, or they can be a complete waste of time.

The strategic planning process you are about to see was designed to be as simple, efficient, and useful as possible. But whether or not the planning processes delivers on those intents will be mostly up to you. As the saying goes, what you put into it (the planning process) will largely determine what you get out of it. Any plan is only as useful, and as practical, as it is well-designed, and actually utilized. It's like a great pair of shoes: it's got to be responsive, practical, workable, and relevant to who you are.

You are therefore encouraged to take as long as you need to in order to complete the following process; however, I encourage you to not rush it and to not take too long. If you rush through the process, you might miss an important opportunity. If you take too long, your enthusiasm will wear thin and you may become disengaged with (quit) the process altogether.

So what is an appropriate pace – somewhere between going too fast or too slow? I recommend that your process take about a month. In the first week you can create your vision and mission statements; in the second week you can assess your subjective well-being; in the third week you can conduct your stakeholder analyses; and in the fourth week you can journal, and chart your way forward by finalizing your contract. I recommend this pacing because I'm assuming that while taking care of these four key areas, you'll also be keeping up with your other work/life demands. If you can clear your schedule, and focus on the process exclusively, it may go a little faster. If you have an especially high tempo in your work or your life, it may take a little longer. But ideally, in about a month from now, you'll have a Well-being Ultimatum strategic plan that is "good to go".

Before you begin this process of creating your plan, I need to make you aware of two key factors that have the potential to either make or break your planning efforts.

The first important factor to remember, is that this entire process will go more smoothly if you engage in it with a trusted friend or coach. Having this support – from one of my certified Centered Well-Being Coaches[1] or your buddy -- will ensure that you

---

[1] If you are interested in training to become a well-being coach certified in my Well-Being Ultimatum system, please see www.drsuziecarmack.com for details on how you can become certified as a coach in my 100-hour certificate program. We would be very happy for you to join us! Some folks take this program so that they can have receive more in-depth training than what is available in this book; they attend the training for their personal knowledge and life application. Others train to become coaches because they want to help others to create their well-being ultimatums, and want to learn the facilitation process that is attached to it. In both cases we welcome you to become certified (although you can still use this process whether you become certified or not). I decided to share this system with the world through this book to help those who are unable to find certification programs in their area to receive the information; and to help those who were considering becoming coaches to understand the program before committing to this training (to be sure it aligns with their beliefs).

have accountability in the process, and will help you to feel that you are not going it alone. It will also be a lot more fun. These are the reasons why social support makes a real difference in behavior change; and why I developed my well-being coach certification process and this model in the first place. I know, in my life, in my research and in my work with clients – that having someone help you makes all of the difference. We healers need help too!

The second factor that you should address in this process, is that while the planning process will take about a month to complete, you really are making a Well-being Ultimatum for a lifetime. I know this is a strong, and bold claim; however, that is the essential point of this entire process. As noted in chapter 2, your Well-being Ultimatum is much like a recovery program. It will take you about a month to understand what is expected of you, and to decide what this understanding will mean for you and your life as you go forward. From there, it is a commitment you will make and remake on a daily basis. This is why we call it a true ultimatum.

WHAT MAKES A GREAT WELL-BEING PLAN?

Plans are meant to be living breathing documents. That said, they can only truly "live and breathe" by being designed, enacted and reworked by people. It is therefore up to us for any plan to work, or not work. If we write a plan, and then ignore it, or if it was created on a false sense of pretenses with regards to "where we are" and/or "where we really want to be" it is doomed to fail before it even begins.

Good plans work best when both "where we want to be" (vision and mission statements) as well as "where we are" (SWOT analysis) are clearly identified. These good plans require a real and sometimes brutal honesty for us to make these identifications, and even more brutal honesty for us to chart from where we are now to where we want to be in a realistic way.

Truly great plans – which is what I hope this Well-being Ultimatum is for you – combine the same sense of honesty, and long-term commitment found in good plans (noted above), with an embedded monitoring and evaluation system. These plans ensure that we not only navigate between where we are now, and where we want to go but that we also track our progress over time. These great plans also respond to changing conditions and/or situational factors that can be "game changers" for our plan; great plans are not stuck in the same set of assumptions.

WBU PLANNING PROCESS – STEP 1
VISION STATEMENT

Many strategic planning processes start with asking you to assess where you are. Rest assure we will get to that. This process however starts with focusing on where you want to be – your "vision of success". Think of this as your North Star which will guide the rest of this (planning) way.

Your creation of your "Vision of your Well-Being Ultimatum Success" comes out of answering any and/or all of the following questions:

1) What does well-being really mean to you?
2) If you had to write a theme for what your life would ideally be, what would it be?

3) Ask 5 people who know you well to say the first three words that they would use to describe you. See if there is a common theme amongst these answers AND see if you like what you hear. The part of you that resists their responses may be your higher voice trying to challenge you to see yourself in bigger and/or better ways.

When I conducted this program with a group recently, the following vision statements emerged. They give you an idea of how short, and specific, a good vision should sound be. You might wish to write a more formal statement than the ones below, but I liked that this particular group created vision statements that sounded like (and in a few cases were) mottos:

Example 1: "Live Long and Prosper"

Example 2 "Make a Difference"

Example 3 "Protect and Serve"

As you can see, we have borrowed from well-known mottos/slogans, and that's OK for this purpose (as long as you don't try to 'borrow' someone else's intellectual property for your next advertising campaign). Having a succinct vision statement (whether or not it is a motto) will summarize what core values you deem important and will give you an overall North Star-type guidance in the steps that follow.

My own vision statement today is "Be the change I wish to see in the world". This of course is borrowed from a well-known quote attributed to Gandhi. For me, my life today is all about helping people to optimize their lives, and I know that this vision depends completely on my own ability and willingness to take my own advice (hence, my writing of this book and my commitment to following its recommendations even as I write and edit).

A few years ago, my vision was "centering the world one person at a time" – which articulated my desire to reach many people in individual ways. Both of my mottos articulate the global health components of my work today; my updated motto indicates how I now "get" that I am of no use to anyone if I don't take my own advice. First.

Interestingly, I found out recently that what I thought was Gandhi's words (my vision statement) is actually a summary of a longer quote, which reads:

> "If we could change ourselves, the tendencies in the world would also change. As a man changes his own nature, so does the attitude of the world change towards him. ... We need not wait to see what others do." - Gandhi

I actually like this interpretation better, because it further articulates my beliefs. It's a little long for a vision statement, but it does summarize the core values I hold dear – which have ramifications in all aspects of my life.

I share this quote here as a gentle reminder to you to be sure that your vision statements (as well as all other elements of your well-being ultimatum plan) are aligned with your "true nature". I want you "not wait to see what others do" but to instead create a Well-being Ultimatum optimization plan that is uniquely yours.

When you have completed your well-being vision statement, place it on the Well-Being Planning worksheet at the end of this chapter.

WBU PLANNING PROCESS – STEP 2
MISSION STATEMENT

In most strategic planning processes, the Mission statement brings the "big dream" of the Vision statement into the "real context" of the real world. According to Forbes Magazine (2015), a company's mission statement should answer the following four questions:

- · What do we do?
- · How do we do it?
- · Whom do we do it for?
- · What value are we bringing?

Your Well-Being Ultimatum mission statement should especially clarify that fourth question – the value proposition of your well-being. What does having, achieving and sustaining do for you and for others? Moreover, what is most important to you with regards to your well-being?

My well-being mission statement is as follows:

Dr. Suzie Carmack is a strategic healer dedicated to promoting health, wellness and well-being. She strategically commits to her own self-care and well-being needs on a daily basis, enjoys time with her family and friends on a weekly basis, and believes in the importance of optimizing quality of life – her own, as well as her family's, her clients', her readers' and her students.

As you can see, it's a little clunky, but it works for me for now—and that's what really matters. It reminds me, when I easily get distracted by projects and/or life events, where my priorities are. It helps me to clarify to myself how I bring my "vision" (for helping the world) into the reality of my life.

Take some time to think through what your mission statement

might include. Feel free to talk with several important people in your life, and ask them to clarify for you what they think you find important.

When you have completed your well-being mission statement, place it on the Well-Being Ultimatum (WBU) planning worksheet at the end of this chapter.

WBU PLANNING PROCESS – STEP 3
SUBJECTIVE WELL-BEING SWOT ANALYSIS

As noted previously, a SWOT analysis is a common component of most strategic planning processes. By clarifying your strengths, weaknesses, opportunities and threats ("SWOT" for short) you can gain a valuable perspective on where you are now, and compare that to your vision and mission statements (where you want to be). The real benefit of a SWOT analysis, is that it gives you efficient perspectives on just how difficult, long, or easy the strategic road between "here and there" will really be.

In order to conduct your SWOT analysis, I encourage you to take the Well-Being Ultimatum surveys (found on my website www.drsuziecarmack.com). These surveys are optional for this Well-Being Ultimatum strategic planning process, but they were chosen to give you perspectives on your five layers (koshas of well-being). Your choice to complete these surveys will also enable my team and I to track potential trends with regards to population well-being.

If you choose to complete these surveys, thank you. I encourage you to take some time to review your answers and to see what the results may say to you. Then answer the questions below. (If you choose not to complete the surveys, please go directly to the questions below).

My unique well-being strengths are:

My weaknesses, which I reframe to myself as vulnerabilities are:

The opportunities I can see for my Well-being Success are:

The threats to my WB I am sensitive to but not afraid of are:

Place the answers to these questions on the WBU worksheet at the end of the chapter.

WBU PLANNING PROCESS – STEP 4
OBJECTIVE WELL-BEING STAKEHOLDER ANALYSIS

"Stakeholders" bring unique and necessary perspectives to any strategic planning process. A stakeholder is someone who has a "stake" in your success. For a company, stakeholders can be both internal (employees, leadership, board) and external (customers, prospective customers, the public). By gaining perspectives from both internal and external stakeholder viewpoints, a company can set a more realistic, and responsive strategic way forward (plan).

This Well-Being Ultimatum strategic planning process similarly asks you to conduct both internal and external stakeholder analysis – starting with this section. In this step, you will complete the external stakeholder analysis, but interviewing people in your life that represent your five key dimensions (Koshas) of well-being. Unlike the first three steps of this strategic planning process, in which you have relied completely on subjective (self-rated) perspectives, this step will offer you an objective view of your well-being. As discussed previously, both subjective and objective perspectives are key to ensuring a full, holistic, and 360 degree perspectives of your well-being.

Here, in this step, I ask that you choose at least one person who represents what each of the Kosha layers mean for you in your life. For example, your doctor, your personal trainer, or even your financial planner, might represent your physical well-being layer. Place the name of each person in the space next to the appropriate layer below.

Physical Well-Being / Functionality Layer _____
Social / Life Force & Balance Layer: _____
Mental / Quality of Life Layer: _____
Spiritual / Meaning and Purpose Layer: _____
Emotional / Happiness Layer: _____

Take time to have a conversation with each of these people (stakeholders) to understand what their perceptions are for your well-being. Ask them to discuss with you how they perceive your well-being currently, and what potential they see for your well-being in the future. Encourage them to be frank with you, so that you can really learn from their suggestions. At the same time, take what you hear in perspective; this is one of the reasons why you are encouraged to talk to at least five people.

After you have interviewed each of these key people, take time to reflect on these stakeholder conversations, and what they mean for you. Then, answer the following questions on page on your WBU planning worksheet at the end of this chapter.

> The Koshas (types of well-being) that are strongest and most viable for me are:

> The Koshas that are weak, drained and/or vulnerable are:

> The opportunities I see to enhance any and/or all of Koshas are:

> The threats I see coming that may compromise my ability to achieve and sustain my Koshas / well-being are...

WBU PLANNING PROCESS – STEP 5
SUBJECTIVE WELL-BEING STAKEHOLDER ANALYSIS

In the last step, we captured and processed your external stakeholders' perspectives. In this step we will conduct an internal stakeholder analysis. This step will ask you to "suspend your disbelief" and imagine that you have a "committee of internal stakeholders" inside your psyche, and that these stakeholders are about to have a board meeting. You are the playwright of this creative exercise and so you get to decide how you take this step on. Be sure to have fun with the following process.

Take some time to imagine that each of the following Kosha layers could be personified. You might imagine each layer as a character, or as a role that you play.

After you have personified each of these Koshas / Well-being dimensions with a name (role, or character), take time to become quiet and meditate /contemplate that these roles have a board meeting to discuss your well-being.

Call the meeting to order by asking each of these board members (roles of your well-being) to clarify what it wants at this board /

bargaining table. Your physical well-being layer might say it wants to eat better, to move more, to sit less, and to have a deeper sense of physical security by taking time this coming year to get your financial house in order. Your spiritual well-being might say it wants to shift the day-day work you are doing because it no longer feels that you are working in ways that fulfill your unique mission/vision. Allow each role to have a moment to speak.

Like any good meeting, it is important that you allow each role to have a voice. Let no role go unheard. At the same time, notice if you have certain roles that are overpowering others. Ensure that by the end of the meeting that all of your roles can agree on a way forward – which will most likely take a bit of negotiation. (If there are particularly difficult 'debates' allow the committee to come up with a plan for how you are going to take on the challenge/impasse over time – much like a company asks a subcommittee to work a particular issue "offline" outside of its regular board meeting).

In my own life I conducted this exercise about a year ago. I won't go into all of the fictitious details, but I can tell you what the experience taught me. It made me realize that certain types of my well-being (certain Koshas) were trying to "run my well-being show". Other roles were surprisingly silent at this meeting. It made me realize that I needed to allow all of my inner stakeholders (well-being roles/koshas) to have a voice, and I needed them all to get along with each other. (One of the reasons you are reading this book right now, is because my Spiritual Well-Being layer said that I needed to write!

Go now to the WBU planning worksheet at the end of this

chapter, and complete this internal stakeholder analysis that is there. Document what each role had to say with regards to the dimensions of your well-being – clarify what each type of well-being sees as an ideal reality. Document what parts of the discussion were difficult and/or easy. Then, allow yourself to journal about what this all means to you, as well as what you have learned from all of the steps thus far.

STEP 6: ANNUAL (LONG-TERM) GOALS

In this step, you put your vision and mission statements up against where your SWOT and stakeholder analyses. You then clarify how you wish to articulate your well-being goals for the next year.

In the WBU planning worksheet at the end of this chapter you will describe what your ideal well-being dimensions will look like in a year. This allows you the freedom to envision the major shifts you want to make over the next year. I have found that many people have an idea of where they want to "take" their well-being, but they find it too daunting to imagine that they could get from here to there in a short / fixed amount of time. A lot can happen in a year. So, by setting your goal against a year timeline, you give yourself some space to make your strategic goals happen. (You can set more long-term goals, at 3- and/or 5-year benchmarks, but I prefer 1-year long-term goals).

This goal list will also serve helpful for your annual evaluation efforts. You can evaluate your success relative to where you have met your goals, where you haven't, and how you have/haven't tracked towards success.

STEP 7: MONTHLY GOALS

One way to begin tackling your annual goals for each dimension of your well-being, found in Step 6, is to break up your steps to get there over seasonal (quarterly) and/or monthly goals. The WBU planning worksheet asks you to take each quarter of the year to focus on your strengths, weaknesses, opportunities and threats.

Another approach to this section, not found on the worksheet, would be to set a goal for each month of the calendar year. For example, you might tackle reorganizing your financial well-being in January; committing to a new fitness regimen in February; taking a course in an activity that is aligned with your spiritual well-being in March, and so on.

It is important to track your monthly success over the course of each month. I like to check in with my monthly goals every 10 days.

STEP 8: WEEKLY GOALS

Your weekly goals are where I believe the Kosha approach to well-being ultimatum comes in the most handy. You simply match each of the Koshas to a different day of the week, and make that your major priority for the day. For example, you might decide that you set your well-being priorities for the day as follows:

Monday: Physical Well-Being
Tuesday: Financial Well-Being
Wednesday: Mental (work/life balance) Well-Being
Thursday: Spiritual (meaning and purpose) Well-Being
Friday: Emotional Well-Being
Saturday: Social Well-Being (time with family/friends)
Sunday: Religious and/or Comprehensive Well-being

This approach does not imply that you will ignore other dimensions of your well-being on alternate days; but it does give you a focus for the day so that you can check in with that well-being dimension and ensure you are not overwhelmed by your long-term commitment to your well-being ultimatum.

You'll also notice that the above daily calendar takes the Koshas "out of order". This is only because many folks spend their weekend time focusing on social and/or religious dimensions of their well-being. You can feel free to change the well-being priority noted for each day to suit your own preferences.

STEP 9: DAILY ACTIONS

As you will see on the WBU worksheet, this section recommends that you address the following self-care needs on a daily basis.

WBU DAILY SELF-CARE CHECKLIST

Medication as per medical directives

Mobility (to not sit too much and to move your major joints)

Exercise (as is appropriate for your age and physical condition)

Nutrition (eat clean in ways appropriate to your energy needs)

Alcohol (Limit, as per medical guidance; drink responsibily)

Sleep (no less than 6 hours per evening)

Detox digitally (with breaks from media and/or email)

Mindfulness (practice self-awareness, gratitude, & meditation)

Non-work endeavors (balance between work & non-work time)

Talk through this list with your buddy and/or coach. Ask them to help you strategize how you will meet each of these objectives. Be honest with them, and yourself, about which areas seem easy for you, and which ones will be difficult. Strategize the ways you will get this list to fit into your day. For example, I practice a digital detox, and my exercise, at the same time.

As you try to determine how you will "make these daily self-care practices actually happen" and fit them into your already-busy calendar, please keep in mind that these recommendations can be adjusted. Although these guidelines follow generally-accepted recommendations with regards to health, wellness and well-being promotion, they may need to be adjusted for your particular life, set of circumstances, and/or health outcomes. For example, if you are a professional athlete, the recommendation to exercise 20 minutes or more per day doesn't work for you during your season; you are exercising much more than that.

My only note of caution, is that I encourage you to be careful. If you find yourself "adjusting the daily plan" and/or "ignoring the daily plan" because of something work-related, and this pattern occurs on a continual basis, then you may need to seek some outside assistance (objective perspectives) on why that is the case (therapist) and/or for strategies to address the issue (well-being coaching with a certified coach).

STEP 10: THE CONTRACT

Ask your well-being buddy, or your coach, to help you to finalize, and then sign your Well-being Ultimatum contract (found at the end of this chapter, and also available on my website, www.drsuziecarmack.com). Place the contract in a frame, in an area where you can see it on a regular basis – to remind you to keep your Well-being Ultimatum with yourself. Let it be an ongoing reminder for your need to a daily commitment to self-care, a weekly commitment to social support, and an ongoing (annual) need for services that will help you to optimize your well-being. These efforts will ensure that you Super Hero aren't just living well; they will help to ensure you can do the Very Important Healing Work you are Called to Do.

Also, be sure to visit our facebook page "Well-Being Ultimatum" to report in on how this well-being ultimatum process went for you. Let us know what worked for you, what was challenging, and what recommendations you would make to others who are about to embark on this process. Also, share your successes – not only to celebrate your hard work but to also encourage others to follow by your example.

I wish you well – and I wish you well-being in all aspects of your life.

See you on the path.

WELL-BEING ULTIMATUM PLANNING WORKSHEET

To me, well-being means…

STEP 1: VISION STATEMENT
My Vision Statement for my life, and my well-being is:

STEP 2: MISSION STATEMENT
My Mission is to:

STEP 3: SUBJECTIVE WELL-BEING SWOT ANALYSIS

According to my completion of the Well-Being Ultimatum surveys (found on www.drsuziecarmack.com), I have discovered the following to be true:

My unique well-being strengths include:

My weaknesses, which I reframe to myself as vulnerabilities are:

The opportunities I can see for my Well-being Success are:

The threats to my WB that I will be sensitive to but not afraid of are:

STEP 4: OBJECTIVE WELL-BENG SWOT ANALYSIS

The following 5 people represent each of my 5 Koshas / Layers (Dimensions) of Well-being:

Physical Well-Being / Functionality Layer _____
Social / Life Force & Balance Layer: _____
Mental / Quality of Life Layer: _____
Spiritual / Meaning and Purpose Layer: _____
Emotional / Happiness Layer: _____

According to my completion of open interviews with each of these people, I have discovered the following to be true:

The Koshas (types of well-being) that are strongest and most viable for me are:

The Koshas that are weak, diffused, drained and/or vulnerable are:

The opportunities I see to enhance any and/or all of my Koshas are:

The threats I see coming that may compromise my ability to achieve and sustain my Koshas / well-being are...

STEP 5: SUBJECTIVE WELL-BEING STAKEHOLDER ANALYSIS

The following 5 Roles that I play in my life represent each of my 5 Koshas / Layers (Dimensions) of Well-being:

Physical Well-Being / Functionality Layer _____
Social / Life Force & Balance Layer: _____
Mental / Quality of Life Layer: _____
Spiritual / Meaning and Purpose Layer: _____
Emotional / Happiness Layer: _____

After taking time (ideally a week or more) to get to know each of these roles, I realize that they each want the following for my well-being:

My Physical (including Financial) Well-Being wants:
My Social Well-Being wants:
My Mental Well-Being wants:
My Spiritual Well-Being wants:
My Emotional Well-Being wants:

When I consider how these wants match up with each other, as well as with my vision and mission statements, I find that... (journal here).

STEP 6: ANNUAL (LONG-TERM) GOALS

After reviewing Parts 1 – 5 above, and further reflection, I declare the following as my Well-Being Ultimatum Goals for the next year:

Physically, my well-being will be experienced as:
Financially, my well-being will be experienced as:
Socially, my well-being will be experienced as:
Mentally, my well-being will be experienced as:

Spiritually, my well-being will be experienced as:
Emotionally, my well-being will be experienced as:

STEP 7: MONTHLY GOALS

In months 1 – 3, I will address the following threats to my well-being:
    To do this, I will lean on the following services:
In months 4 – 6, I will work to develop opportunities for my well-being
    To do this, I will lean on the following services:
In months, 7 – 9, I will celebrate my well-being strengths by:
    To do this, I will lean on the following services:
In months, 10 – 12, I will have transformed my challenges by:
    To do this, I will lean on the following services:

STEP 8: WEEKLY PRACTICES

I will take care of my well-being dimensions weekly by:

    Focusing on Physical Well-Being Monday by:
    Focusing on Financial Well-Being Tuesday by:
    Focusing on Mental Well-Being Wednesday by:
    Focusing on Spiritual Well-Being Thursday by:
    Focusing on Emotional Well-Being Friday by:
    Focusing on Social Well-Being Saturday by:
    Focusing on Religious and/or Comprehensive Well-Being Sunday by:

I will check in with my Well-Being Coach / Buddy _____

STEP 9: DAILY PRACTICES:
See the WBU contract for a detailed listing of the daily practices.

STEP 10: THE WELL-BEING ULTIMATUM CONTRACT

I _____, recognizing that a sound mind, body, heart, spirit and life are all of vital importance to me, my family, my friends, and those I heal in my work as a _____ make this Well-Being Ultimatum with myself.

___ Today, I would describe my well-being as: _____
My well-being is currently challenged by _____
In the next year, I would like to improve my well-being: by:_____.___
I will know my efforts over the next year are successful when: _____

___ I recognize that I deserve to enjoy a good life, and to live in ways that are good for me.

___ I welcome the longevity, prosperity, and overall quality of life that results when I balance my desire to heal others with my own personal needs for self-care, social support & services.

___ I recognize that my health, my wellness, and my well-being can no longer afford to be ignored, dysfunctional or less than optimal. I seek to prevent, or combat, the effects of compassion fatigue, burnout, and other disorders that occur when my energy is drained.

___ I agree to regularly check in with my buddy / coach to monitor and evaluate my progress.

SELF-CARE
On a Daily Basis, I will commit to the following Self-Care practices
1) I will take all medications as directed by my doctor.
2) I will limit my sitting behavior during the workday by:_____
3) I will move my body for at least 20 minutes per day by: _____
4) I will aim to get between ___ and ___ hours of sleep (>6.5 hrs).
5) I will eat well more than I do not, as needed for my activity level
6) I will limit my use of alcohol, and will drink responsibly.
7) I will take at least 10 min. per day to practice mindfulness (which may or may not be combined with movement and/or stillness).
8) I will digitally detox daily by (e.g. limiting screen time after 9 pm; limiting check-ins on social media, and/or: _____)
9) I will spend time every day engaged in non-work activities such as: _____
10) I will commit to my weekly well-being goals on a daily basis as follows:
    Mondays (Physical Well-Being)
    Tuesdays (Financial Well-Being)
    Wednesdays (Mental (Work/Life Balance) Well-being
    Thursdays (Spiritual (Career/Meaning and Purpose) Well-being
    Fridays (Emotional (Happiness) Well-Being)
    Saturdays (Social Well-Being)
    Sunday (Comprehensive or Religious Well-Being + Goal Check)

SOCIAL SUPPORT
In addition to making a point weekly to ensure that I spend quality, undistracted time with my family and friends, I will also take time throughout the week and the month to catch up with those who are near and dear to my heart.

SERVICES
I agree to allow myself to be vulnerable enough to admit and recognize when I need help from a variety of services, which may include but are not limited to: legal, financial, physical, medical, stress management, and/or any other key service area that will help to enhance, support and "back up" my well-being.

I look forward to optimizing my mind, body, life and spirit from this day forward.

SIGNED: _____ Date _____
WITNESS _____ Date:: _____
(Buddy or Certified Centered Well-Being © Coach)

Thank you for reading Well-Being Ultimatum!

If you found the book helpful, I would be humbled and honored for you to recommend it to your friends and colleagues on social media and/or in your real life. Because after all, we Super Heroes need to stick together.

I wish you peace, joy and love.

-- Suzie

Please visit my website to learn more about:

Daily "Well-Being Ultimatum" breaks – Join me every workday for a "centering" practice for your well-being. In only 15 minutes, you'll learn gentle movements, active mindfulness and positive intentions can improve your well-being. (New sessions posted every day!)

Monthly Well-Being Ultimatum Seminars
Join me for a live stream class once monthly – either live or by download. Each month we will discuss and explore a new Well-Being Ultimatum dimension or theme. I'd love to hear your questions too!

Coach and Teacher Certificate Program
I enjoy training Well-Being Coaches, Yoga Teachers and Pilates teachers through my internationally-recognized program. You can join us to learn how to share Well-Being Ultimatum methods with others!

Research Opportunities

and

Surveys to Assess and Track Subjective and Objective Well-being

www.DrSuzieCarmack.com.

REFERENCES

Angner, E. (2009). Subjective Well-being (unpublished) – University of Alabama.

"Burnout." Merriam-Webster.com. Merriam-Webster, n.d. Web. 16 Aug. 2015. <http://www.merriam-webster.com/dictionary/burnout>.

Carmack, S. (2014). Making Sense of Well-Being: Mixed-method study applying sense-making theory to explore the role of communication competence and social support in physical, emotional, mental and comprehensive well-being. (Doctoral Dissertaiton). George Mason University. http://digilib.gmu.edu.

Collier, M. J. (2005). Theorizing cultural identifications: Critical updates and continuing evolution. In W. B. Gudykunst (Ed.), *Theorizing about intercultural communication* (pp. 235-256). Thousand Oaks, CA: Sage.

Collier, M. J. (2009). Cultural identity theory. In S. W. Littlejohn & K. A. Foss (Eds.), *Encyclopedia of communication theory* (Vol. 1, pp. 260-262). Thousand Oaks, CA: Sage.

"Compassion Fatigue." (n.d.) *Medical Dictionary.* (2009). Retrieved August 16 2015 from http://medical-dictionary.thefreedictionary.com/compassion+fatigue

Dossey, L. (1982). Space, Time and Medicine, Boulder, CO: Shambhala.

Forbes Magazine (2015), Answer Four Questions to Get a Great Mission Statement. Retrieved August 11, 2015 from http://www.forbes.com/sites/patrickhull/2013/01/10/answer-4-questions-to-get-a-great-mission-statement/.

Fortgang (1999) #401 from Innovative Leader Volume 8, Number 5 May 1999 retrieved July 13, 2015 from http://www.winstonbrill.com/bril001/html/article_index/articles/401-450/article401_body.html.

Glanz, K., Lewis, F.M. and Rimer, B.K. (1997a) Linking theory, research and practice. In Glanz, K., Lewis, F.M. and Rimer, B.K. (eds), Health Behavior and Health Education: Theory, Research and Practice, 2nd edn. Jossey-Bass, San Francisco, CA, pp. 19–35.

"Health Disparity" Centers for Disease Control Website. Retrieved August 11, 2015 http://www.cdc.gov/minorityhealth/.

Jackson, R. L. (1999). *The negotiation of cultural identity: Perceptions of European and African Americans.* Westport, CT: Praeger.

Jonas, Wayne B. ; O'connor, Francis G. ; Deuster, Patricia ; Peck, Jonathan ; Shake, Caron ; Frost, Stephen S. (2010). Why Total Force Fitness? *Military Medicine*, 175(8S), pp.6-13

"Koshas" (n.d.) Radiant Light Yoga (2015). Retrieved August 11, 2015 from http://radiantlightyoga.com/content/articles/the-koshas/

Lombardo, B., Eyre, C., (Jan 31, 2011) "Compassion Fatigue: A Nurse's Primer" OJIN: The Online Journal of Issues in Nursing Vol. 16, No. 1, Manuscript 3.

McGonigal, K. (2013) How to Make Stress Your Friend (Video / Ted Talk). http://www.ted.com/talks/kelly_mcgonigal_how_to_make_stress_your_friend/citations

Smith, P. (2015) Compassion Fatigue website: www.compassionfatigue.org.

Stroka (2015) The interaction between "yin" and "yang": "Sympathetic Nervous System (SNS)" – "Parasympathetic Nervous System (PNS)" Retrieved August 11, 2015 from http://heartattacknew.com/faq/what-is-the-relationship-between-stress-and-heart-attacks/

Ting-Toomey, S. (1999). *Communicating across cultures*. New York, NY: Guilford Press.

"Ultimatum." *Merriam-Webster.com*. Merriam-Webster, n.d. Web. 16 Aug. 2015. <http://www.merriam-webster.com/dictionary/ultimatum>.

"Wellness Wheel" (2015). University of Utah Center for Student Wellness. Retrieved August 11, 2015. http://wellness.utah.edu/wellness-wheel.php

ADDITIONAL READING / RESOURCES / INSIGHTS

Albrecht, T. L., & Adelman, M. B. (1987). Communicating social support: A theoretical perspective. In T. L. Albrecht & M. B. Adelman (Eds.), *Communicating social support* (pp. 18–39). Newbury Park, CA: Sage.

Albrecht, T. L., & Adelman, M. B. (1987). Rethinking the relationship between communication and social support: An introduction. In T. L. Albrecht & M. Adelman (Eds.), Communicating social support (pp. 13–16). Newbury Park, CA: Sage.

Apker, J., Ford, W. S. Z., & Fox, D. H. (2003). Predicting nurse's organizational and professional identification: The effect of nursing roles, professional autonomy, and supportive communication. Nursing Economics, 21, 226–232.

Ancona, D. (2012). Sensemaking: Framing and Acting in the Unknown; as seen in Snook, S; Nohria, N; Khurana (2012). *The Handbook for Teaching Leadership: Knowing, Doing and Being*. Sage Publications.

Andrews, F. M. & Withey, S.B. (1976). *Social indicators of Well-Being: America's perception of life quality*. New York: Plenum Press.

Allen, (2009). Measures of Health Literacy: Workshop Summary. Institute of Medicine (US) Roundtable on Health Literacy. Washington (DC): National Academies Press (US); 2009.

Angner, E. (2011). The Evolution of Eupathics: The Historical Roots of Subjective Measures of Well-Being *International Journal of Wellbeing*, Vol. 1, No. 1, pp. 4-41. Retrieved from http://papers.ssrn.com/sol3/papers.cfm?abstract_id=799166

APA (2013).http://www.apa.org/pi/about/publications/caregivers/ practicesettings/assessment/tools/patient-health.aspx

Argyle, M. (2001) *The Psychology of Happiness*. Routledge.

Bansler, J., & Havn, E. (2006). Sensemaking in technology-use mediation: Adapting groupware technology in organizations. *Computer Supported Cooperative Work,15*(1), 55–91.

Baum, F. (1995). Researching Public Health: Behind the qualitative-quantiative methodological debate. *Social Science and Medicine, 40*: 459 – 468.

Bauman, A., Ainsworth, B. E., Sallis, J. F., Hagströmer, M., Craig, C. L., Bull, F. C., & Sjöström, M. (2011). The Descriptive Epidemiology of Sitting: A 20-Country Comparison Using the International Physical Activity Questionnaire (IPAQ). *American Journal Of Preventive Medicine, 41*(2), 228-235. doi:10.1016/j.amepre.2011.05.003

Becchetti, L., Castriota, S., & Giuntella, O. (2006). *The Effects of Age and JoB Protection on the Welfare Costs of Inflation and Unemployment: a Source of ECB anti-inflation bias?* Centre for Economic and International Studies (CEIS) Working Paper No. 245.

Becchetti, L., Castriota, S., & Londoño Bedoya, D.A. (2007). *Climate, Happiness and the Kyoto protocol: someone does not like it hot.* Centre for Economic and International Studies (CEIS) Working Paper No. 247.

Beiser, M. (1974). Composites and Correlates of Mental Well-Being. *Journal of Health & Social Behavior, 15*, 320-327.

Ben- Shahar, T. (2007). *Happier: Learn the Secrets to Daily Joy and Lasting Fulfillment.* New York, McGraw-Hill

Berger, C. R., Calabrese, R. J. (1975). Some Exploration in Initial Interaction and Beyond:Toward a Developmental Theory of Communication. *Human Communication Research*, 1, 99–112.

Bergstrom, A., Pisani, A., Tenet, V., Wolk, A., & Adami, H. O. (2001). Overweight as an avoidable cause of cancer in Europe. *International Journal of Cancer, 91*, 421–430 as cited in Ricciardi, R. (2005). Sedentarism: a concept analysis. *Nursing Forum, 40*(3), 79-87.

Blanchflower, D.G. (2008). International Evidence on Well-being. IZA DP No. 3354. Institute for the Study of Labor, Bonn Blanchflower, D.G. (2007). Is Well-Being U-Shaped Over the Life Cycle? NBER Working Paper No. 12935. Cambridge, Mass: National Bureau of Economic Research.

Blazer, D. G. (1982). Social support and mortality in an elderly community population. *American Journal of Epidemiology, 115*, 684–694.

Broadhead, W. E., Kaplan, B. H., James, S. A., Wagner, E. H., Schoenbach, V. J., Grimson, R., Heyden, S., Tibblin, G., & Gehlbach, S. H. (1983). The epidemiologic evidence for a relationship between social support and health. *American Journal of Epidemiology, 117*, 521–537.

Brickman, P., Coates, D, a& Janoff-Bulman.J. (1978). Lottery Winners and Accident Victims: Is Happiness Relative? *Journal of Personality and Social Psychology* 36(8): 917-927.

Brown, K.; Ryan, R. (2003). The benefits of being present: Mindfulness and its role in psychological well-being. *Journal of Personality and Social Psychology*, 84, 822-848.

Bruni, L.& Porta, P.L. (2007). Introduction. In Luigino Bruni and Pier Luigi Porta, eds. *Handbook on the Economics of Happiness*. Cheltenham, UK:Edward Elgar.

Caldwell, K., Harrison, M., Adams, M., Quin, R., & Greeson, J. (2010). Developing mindfulness in college students through movement-based courses: Effects on self-regulatory self-efficacy, mood, stress, and sleep quality. *Journal of American College Health*, 58, 433-442.

Canary, D. J., Cunningham, E. M., & Cody, M. J. (1988). Goal types, gender, and locus of control in the management of interpersonal conflict. Communication Research, 15, 426–446.

Canary, D.J., & Lakey, S. G. (2006). Managing conflict in a competent manner: A mindful look at events that matter. In J. G. Oetzel & S. Ting-Toomey (Eds.), The Sage handbook of conflict communication (pp. 185–210). Thousand Oaks, CA: Sage.

Carmody, J., & Baer, R. A. (2008). Relationships between mindfulness practice and levels of mindfulness, medical and psychological symptoms and well-being in a mindfulness-based stress reduction program. *Journal of Behavioral Medicine, 31*(1), 23-33.

Cassell, J. (1976). The contribution of the social environment to host resistance. *American Journal of Epidimiology, 104*, 107–123.

Chavez, C., Backett-Milburn, K., Parry, O., & Platt, S. (2005). Understanding and Researching Wellbeing: Its usage in different disciplines and potential for health research and health promotion. *Health Education Journal.* Sage Publications. Retrieved January 2, 2013 from: http://hej.sagepub.com/content/64/1/70

Chen, Y., & Feeley, T. (2012). Enacted Support and Well-Being: A Test of the Mediating Role of Perceived Control. *Communication* Studies, 63(5), 608-625. doi:10.1080/10510974.2012.674619

Chopra, P. K., & Kanji, G. K. (2010). Emotional intelligence: A catalyst for inspirational leadership and management excellence. *Total Quality Management & Business Excellence, 21*(10), 971-1004. doi:10.1080/14783363.2010.487704

Campbell, A.; Converse, P.E.; & Rogers, W.L. (1976). *The quality of American Life: Perceptions, Evaluations and Satisfactions.* New York: Russell Sage Foundation.

Centers for Disease Control (2013) The Rapid Assessment of Physical Activity. Retrieved from Http://depts.washington.edu/hprc/rapa.

Clarke, P. N. & Yaros, P. S. (1988). Research blenders: Commentary and response. *Nursing Science Quarterly, (1)*, 147 – 149.

Cobb, S. (1976). Social support as a moderator of life stress. *Psychosomatic Medicine, 38*, 300–314.

Cohen, S., Kamarck, T., & Mermelstein, R. (1983). A Global Measure of Perceived stress. *Journal of Health and Social Behavior, 24,* 385-396.

Cohen, S. (1988). Psychosocial models of the role of social support in the etiology of physical disease. *Health Psychology, 7*, 269–297.

Conceico, P. & Bandura, R. (2008) Measuring Well-Being: A summative review of the literature United Nations Development Program, Development Studies Research Papers. December 12, 2012 from: *web.undp.org/.../subjective_wellbeing_conceicao_bandura.pdf.*

Cooley, R. E. & Roach, D. A. (1984). A conceptual framework. In R. N. Bostrom (Ed.), *Competence in communication: A multidisciplinary approach* (pp. 11-32). Beverly Hills, CA: Sage. Colangelo, L. (2011). Course website ttp://www.austincc.edu/colangelo/1318/interpersonalcommunicationcompetence.

Crisp, R. (2006). Hedonism reconsidered. *Philosophy and Phenomenological Research, 73(3),* 619-645.

Cummins, R. A. (2010). Fluency disorders and life quality: Subjective wellbeing vs. health-related quality of life. *Journal Of Fluency Disorders, 35*(3), 161-172. doi:10.1016/j.jfludis.2010.05.009

Cunningham, Stanley B. (1992). "Intrapersonal Communication: A Review and Critique," *Communication Yearbook #15,* (Newbury Park, CA: Sage Publications), pp. 597-620.

Cupach, W. R., & Canary, D. J. (2000). Competence in Interpersonal conflict. Prospect Heights, IL: Waveland. Dankoski, M. (2007). What's Love Got to Do With It? Couples, Illness, and MFT. *Journal Of Couple & Relationship Therapy, 6*(1/2), 31.

Deaton, A. (2008). Income, Health, and Well-Being around the World: Evidence from the Gallup World Poll. *Journal of Economic Perspectives* 22(2): 53-72.

DeHaes, J. C.; Pennink, B. J. W.; & Welvaart, K. (1987). The Distinction Between Affect and Cognition. *Social Indicators Research, 19* 367-378.

Deci, E. L. & Ryan, R. M. (2008) Self-Determination Theory: A Macrotheory of Human Motivation,Development, and Health. *Canadian Psychology 49* (3), 182–185

Dervin, B. (1976a). Strategies for dealing with human information needs: Information or communication? *Journal of Broadcasting, 20(3),* 324-351.

Dervin, B. (1983). An overview of sense-making research: Concepts, methods and results. Paper presented at the annual meeting of the *International Communication Association.* Dallas, TX.

Dervin, B. (1992). From the mind's eye of the user: The sense-making qualitativequantitative methodology. In Glazier, J. and Powell, R. R. *Qualitative research in information management* (p. 61-84). Englewood, CA: Libraries Unlimited

Dervin, B. (1996). Given a context by any other name: Methodological tools for taming the unruly beast. Keynote paper, *ISIC 96: Information Seeking in Context.* 1–23.

Dervin, B. (1999). Chaos, order, and Sense-Making: A proposed theory for information design. In R. Jacobson, eds. *Information design.* Cambridge, MA: MIT Press, 35- 57.

Dervin, B., & Nilan, M. (1986). Information needs and uses. *Annual Review of Information Science and Technology, 21,* 3–33.

Dervin, B. (1999). On studying information seeking methodologically: The implications of connecting metatheory to method. *Information Processing and Management, 35*(6), 727–750.

Dervin, B. (2003). Given a context by any other name: Methodological tools for taming the unruly beast. In B. Dervin, L. Foreman-Wernet, & E. Lauterbach (Eds.), *Sensemaking methodology reader: Selected writings of Brenda Dervin* (pp. 111–132). Cresskill, NJ: Hampton Press.

Dervin, B. (2003). *Information Design*. Chaos, Order, and Sense-Making: A ProposedTheory for Information Design. *Volume 4*. Pages: 325-340. *Issue: 3/4.*

Dervin, B. (2005). Libraries reaching out with health information to vulnerable populations: Guidance from research on information seeking and use. *Journal of the Medical Library Association* 94 (4): S74-S80.

Dervin, B. (2008). Interviewing as dialectical practice: Sense-Making Methodology as exemplar. Presented at *International Association of Media and Communication Research (IAMCR) Meeting,* Stockholm, Sweden: 20–25.

Dervin, B., Fisher, K. E., Durrance, J., Ross, C., Savolainen, R., & Solomon, P. (2005). Reports of the demise of the "user" have been greatly exaggerated: Dervin's sensemaking and the methodological resuscitation of the user-looking backwards, looking forward. *Proceedings of the American Society for Information Science and Technology, 42*(1).

Diener, E. (2000). Subjective Well-Being. The Science of Happiness and a Proposal for a National Index. *American Psychologist, 55* (1), 34-43.

Diener, E.; Suh, E. (1997). Measuring quality of life: economic, social, and subjective indicators. *Social Indicators Research* 40,189-216.

Diener, E., Emmons, R. A., Larsen, R. J., & Griffin, S. (1985). The Satisfaction with Life scale. *Journal of Personality Assessment, 49* (1), 71-75.

Diener, E., Suh, E.M, Lucas, R.E. & Smith, H.L. (1999). Subjective Well-Being: Three Decades of Progress. *Psychological Bulletin,* 125 (2), 276-302.

Diener, E., & Suh, E.M. (1997). Measuring quality of life: Economic, social and subjective indicators. *Social Indicators Research, 40* (1-2), 189-216.

Diener, E. (1994). Assessing Subjective Well-Being: Progress and Opportunities. *Social Indicators Research,* 31 (2), 103-157.

Diener, E. (1984). Subjective Well-Being. *Psychologial Bulletin.* 95, 542-575.

Dumith, S. C., Hallal, P. C., Reis, R. S., & Kohl, H. W. (2011). Worldwide prevalence of physical inactivity and its association with human development index in 76 countries. *Preventive Medicine, 53*(1/2), 24-28. doi:10.1016/j.ypmed.2011.02.017.

Dupuy, H. J. (1977). The General Well-being Schedule. In McDowell, C Newell (Eds.), *Measuring health: a guide to rating scales and questionnaire* (2nd ed) (pp. 206- 213). USA: Oxford University Press.

Easterlin, R. (2004). *The Economics of Happiness.* Daedalus 133(2): 26-33.

Easterlin, R. (2003). Explaining Happiness. Inaugural Articles by members of the National Academy of Sciences. PNAS 100(19): 11176–11183.

Eid, M., and Larsen, R. J. (2008). *The Science of Subjective Well-being* New York: The Guilford Press.

Espinoza, S.; Posegate, A.; Rowan, K.; Wilson, K.; Zhao, X.; & Maibach, E. (2012) Television weathercasters as environmental science communicators. In D. Rigling Gallagher (Ed.) *Environmental Leadership Reference Handbook.* Thousand Oaks, CA: SAGE. p. 411-19.

Ewin, J. (2000). *Nutritional Therapy.* Elementary Books Limited, Shaftesbury, Dorset, http://www.researchsurveys.co.za/research-papers/pdf/02_gini.pdf

Extremera, N., Ruiz-Aranda, D., Pineda-Galán, C., & Salguero, J. M. (2011). Emotional intelligence and its relation with hedonic and eudaimonic well-being: A prospective study. *Personality & Individual Differences, 51*(1), 11-16. doi:10.1016/j.paid.2011.02.029

Floyd, K. (2001). Human Affection Exchange: I. Reproductive Probability as a Predictor of Men's Affection with Their Sons. *Journal Of Men's Studies, 10*(1), 39-50.

Floyd, K., & Morr, M. (2003). Human Affection Exchange: VII. Affectionate Communication in the Sibling/Spouse/ Sibling-in-Law Triad. *Communication Quarterly, 51*(3), 247-261.

Floyd, K., & Deiss, D. M. (2012). Better health, better lives: The bright side of affection. In T. J. Socha & M. Pitts (Eds.), *The positive side of interpersonal communication* (pp. 127-142). New York: Peter Lang Publishing.

Folkman, S. (2008). The case for positive emotions in the stress process. *Anxiety Stress Coping, 21*(1), 3-14.

Frey, B,S., & Stutzer, A. (2000). Happiness, Economics and Institutions. The Economic Journal 110 (October): 918-938.

Frisch, M. (2006). *Quality of life therapy: Applying a life satisfaction approach to positive psychology and cognitive therapy.* Hoboken, NJ

Froh, J.J. (2006). Counting blessings in early adolescents: A experimental study of gratitude and subjective well-being. *Journal of School Psychology, 46* (2008) 213– 233. Gallup-Healthways, http://www.well-beingindex.com/methodology.asp, retrieved April 2, 2013.

Gasper, D. (2007). Conceptualizing Human Needs and Well-being; In, Gough, I. and McGregor, J. A. (Eds.) *Researching Well-being in Developing Countries: From Theory to Research.* pp. 47-70. Cambridge, UK: Cambridge University Press

Gioia, D. A. (2006). On Weick: An appreciation. *Organization Studies, 27*(11), 1709–1721.

Ghorbanshiroudi S, Khalatbari J, Salehi M, Bahari S, Keikhayfarzaneh M. (2011). The relationship between emotional intelligence and life satisfaction and determining their communication skill test effectiveness. *Indian Journal Of Science & Technology* [serial online]. November 2011;4(11):1560-1564. Available from: Academic Search Complete, Ipswich, MA. Accessed June 25, 2013.

Lindsey, E. W., Cremeens, P. R., Colwell, M. J., & Caldera, Y. M. (2009). The Structure of Parent–Child Dyadic Synchrony in Toddlerhood and Children's Communication Competence and Self-control. Social Development, 18(2), 375-396. doi:10.1111/j.1467-9507.2008.00489.x

Gilchrist, E. S., & Weinstein, S. D. (November, 2010). Examining Relational Health Communication Competence and Social Support Among Parents of Children Living with Severe and Persistent Mental Illness: An additional multivariate test of the Relational Health Communication Competence Model. Paper presented at the National Communication Association convention, San Francisco, Health Communication Division.

Gilchrist, E. S., & Query, J. L. (April, 2010). Using the relational health communication competence model to examine the relationships of communication competence and social support to job burnout and job engagement of assisted living facility employees. Paper presented at the Central States Communication Association convention, Cincinnati, Health Communication Division.

Giatti, C., Rodrigues, & Barreto, (2012) Reliability of the MacArthur scale of subjective social status - Brazilian Longitudinal Study of Adult Health (ELSA-Brasil) *BMC Public Health* 2012, **12**:1096 doi:10.1186/1471-2458-12-1096 Retrieved June 9, 2013 from: http://www.biomedcentral.com/1471-2458/12/1096

Hallett, V. (2012) centeredbeing: Getting exercise at your desk. *Washington Post*: September 11, 2012 http://articles.washingtonpost.com/2012-09-11/lifestyle/35496943_1_chairs-movement-desk

Helliwell, John F. (2003). How's life? Combining individual and national variables to explain subjective well-being. Economic Modelling 20(2): 331-360.

Henriques, G.H. (2011) http://www.psychologytoday.com/blog/theoryknowledge/ 201112/kahneman-well-being-and-domains-consciousness

Hood, C., & Carruthers, C. (2007). Enhancing leisure experience and developing resources: The Leisure and Well-Being model, Part II. Therapeutic Recreation Journal, 41, 298-325.

Isen, A, M., Daubman, K.A., & Nowicki, G.P. (1987). Positive affect facilitates creative problem solving. *Journal of Personality and Social Psychology, 56(6),* 1122-1131

Joseph, S., & Linley, P. (2006). Positive therapy: A meta-theory for positive psychological practice. New York: Routledge.

Judge, T. A., & Hulin, C. L. (1990). *Job satisfaction as a reflection of disposition: A multiple source casual analysis* (CAHRS Working Paper #90-22). Ithaca, NY: Cornell University, School of Industrial and Labor Relations, Center for Advanced Human Resource Studies. http://digitalcommons.ilr.cornell.edu/cahrswp/387

Kabat-Zinn, J. (2003). Mindfulness-based interventions in context: Past, present, and future. *Clinical Psychology: Science and Practice, 10,* 144-156.

Kahneman, D, & Krueger, A.B. (2006). Developments in the Measurement of Subjective Well-Being. *Journal of Economic Perspectives 20* (1): 3–24.

Kahneman, (2010). The Riddle of Experience Vs. Memory. Ted
Talks:http://www.ted.com/talks/daniel_kahneman_the_riddle_of_experience_vs_memory.
html. Retrieved December 12, 2012.

Kar, S., Thakur, J., Virdi, N., Jain, S., & Kumar, R. (2010). Risk factors for cardiovascular
diseases: is the social gradient reversing in northern India?. *The National Medical Journal of
India, 23*(4), 206-209.

Kazak, A. (2006). Pediatric Psychosocial Preventative Health Model (PPPHM): research,
practice, and collaboration in pediatric family systems medicine. *Families, Systems & Health:
The Journal of Collaborative Family Healthcare, 24*(4), 381-395.

Keaten, J., & Kelly, L. (2008). Emotional Intelligence as a Mediator of Family
Communication Patterns and Reticence. *Communication Reports, 21*(2), 104-116.
doi:10.1080/08934210802393008

Keune, P. M., & Forintos, D. (2010). Mindfulness Meditation: A Preliminary Study on
Meditation Practice During Everyday Life Activities and its Association with Well-Being.
Psihologijske Teme / Psychological Topics, 19(2), 373-386.

Keller, S. (2004). Welfare and the achievement of goals. *Philosophical Studies* 121, 27- 41.

Klein, G., Moon, B. and Hoffman, R.F. (2006a). Making sense of sensemaking I: alternative
perspectives. *IEEE Intelligent Systems*, 21(4), 70–73.

Klein, G., Moon, B. and Hoffman, R.F. (2006b). Making sense of sensemaking Ii: a
macrocognitive model. *IEEE Intelligent Systems*, 21(5), 88–92

Kort B., Reilly, R. & Picard R. (2001) An affective model of interplay between emotions and
learning: reengineering educational pedagogy—building a learning companion, in: T.
Okamoto, R. Hartley, Kinshuk & J. P. Klus (Eds) *Proceedings
of the IEEE International Conference on Advanced Learning Technology: Issues,Achievements and
Challenges* (Madison, WI, IEEE Computer Society), 43–48.

Kreps, G. L. (2009). Applying Weick's model of organizing to health care and health
promotion: Highlighting the central role of health communication. *Patient Education and
Counseling, 74*, 347-355.

Kreps G. L. (1988) Relational communication in health care. *Southern Speech Communication
Journal.* 53(4):344-359.

Kreps, G. L., Bonaguro, E. W., & Query, J. L. (1998). The history and development of the
field of health communication. In L. D. Jackson & B. K. Duffy (Eds.), *Health communication
research: A guide to developments and directions* (pp. 1–15).

Westport, CT: Greenwood Press Kreps, G.L., & Neuhauser, L. (2010). New Directions in
Ehealth Communication: Opportunities and challenges. *Patient   Education and Counseling,*
78, pp. 329-336.

Kreps, G. L., & Thornton, B. C. (1984). *Health Communication: Theory and practice.* New York:
Longman.

Kroenke, K., Spitzer, R,L, Williams, J.B. (2001). The PHQ-9: Validity of a brief depression measure. Journal of General Internal Medicine, 16:603-613.

Levine, J. A. (2010) Health Chair Reform: Your Chair: Comfortable but deadly. *Diabetes* November 2010 (59)11, pp. 2715-2716.

Liang, J. (1985). A Structural Integration of the Affect Balance Scale and the Life Satifaction Index A. *Journal of Gerontology, 40,* 552-561.

Lyubomirsky, S., & Lepper, H. (1999). A measure of subjective happiness: Preliminary reliability and construct validation. *Social Indicators Research, 46,* 137-155. The original publication is available at www.springerlink.com.

Ma, J. & Latham, D. (2013). Interacting with health information for self-care: A pilot study exploring undergraduates' health information literacy. iConference 2013 Proceedings (pp. 793-796). doi:10.9776/13390.

MacArthur Network on SES & Health (2007) The MacArthur Scale of Subjective Social Status. Retrieved April 28, 2013 from http://www.macses.ucsf.edu/research/psychosocial/subjective.php.
Makoul, G., Clayman, M., Lynch, E., Thompson, J. (2009). Four Concepts of Health in America: Results of National Surveys. *Journal of Health Communication, 14*: 3 –14.

Matthews, C., George, S., Moore, S., Bowles, H., Blair, A., Park, Y., & Schatzkin, A. (2012). Amount of time spent in sedentary behaviors and cause-specific mortality in US adults. *American Journal Of Clinical Nutrition, 95*(2), 437-445. doi:10.3945/ajcn.111.019620.

McDowell, I. (2006). *Measuring health: a guide to rating scales and questionnaires* (3rd ed.). USA: Oxford University Press.

McDowell, I. And Newell, C. (1996). *Measuring health.* New York: Oxford University Press.

McGillivray, M. (2007). Human Well-being: Issues, Concepts and Measures. In Mark Q McGillivray, ed. *Human Well-Being: Concept and Measurement.* Basingstoke,UK: Palgrave MacMillan.

McGillivray, M., & Clarke, M. (2006). Human Well-being: Concepts and Measures. In Mark McGillivray and Matthew Clarke, eds. *Understanding Human Well-Being.* Basingstoke: Palgrave MacMillan.

Mehnert, T., Krauss, H.H., Nadler, R., & Boyd, M. (1990).
Correlates of Life Satisfaction in Those with Disabling Conditions. *Rehabilitation Psychology* 35(1): 3-17.

Miller, K. (1995). *Organizational Communication: Approaches and processes.* Wadsworth Publishing: Belmont, CA.
Montgomery, G. H., Erblich, J., DiLorenzo, R., Bovbjerg, D. H. (2003) Family and friends with disease: their impact on perceived risk. *Preventative Medicine, 37*: 242-9.

National Institutes of Health, 2013 website: http://www.nih.gov/clearcommunication/"The Pink Book" National Cancer Institute, 2008, accessed April 27, 2013

NWIA (National Wellness Institute of Australia (2012). Website:

http://nwia.idwellness.org/

Neighmond, P. (2011) Sitting All Day: Worse for You Than You Might Think. www.npr.org. http://www.npr.org/2011/04/25/135575490/sitting-all-day-worsefor-you-than-you-Might-think.

Nelson, D. B., & Nelson, K. W. (2003). Emotional Intelligence Skills: Significant Factors in Freshmen Achievement and Retention.

Neuhauser, L. (2010). Creating and implementing large-scale parenting education programs: Bridging research, decision-making and practice. In Bammer, G., Michaux, A., and Sanson, A. (Eds.) Bridging the "Know-Do" Gap: Knowledge Brokering to Improve Child Well-Being. *Australian National University Press.*

Neuhauser, L., & Kreps, G. (2011) Participatory Design and Artificial Intelligence: Strategies to improve health communication for diverse audiences. Paper presented to the AAAI Spring Symposium 2011. Retrieved from http://www.informatik.unitrier.de/~ley/db/conf/aaaiss/ aaaiss2011-1.html.

Neuhauser, L., Rothschild, B., Graham, C., Ivey, S., & Konishi, S. Participatory Design of Mass Health Communication in Three Languages for Seniors and People with Disabilities on Medicaid. *American Journal of Public Health.* Pub. Oct.15, 2009.

Neuhauser, L. & Kreps, G. (2011). Participatory Design and Artificial Intelligence: Strategies to improve health communication for diverse audiences. Paper presented to the AAAI Spring Symposium 2011. Retrieved from http://www.informatik.unitrier. de/~ley/db/conf/aaaiss/aaaiss2011-1.html.

Oswald, A. J. (1997). Happiness and Economic Performance. *Economic Journal* 107(5): 1815–31.

Ostrow, R. (2005). What wellbeing really means. Retrieved 12/10/12 from: NewsBank. http://140.234.0.9:8080/EPSessionID =e8847763ad982bdeaaaf065b4f53431/EPHost=infoweb.newsbank.com/EPPath/iwsearch/ we/InfoWeb?p_product=AWNB&p_theme=aggregated5&p_action=doc&p_docid=1095A 8ED34FCD43F&p_docnum=2&p_queryname=1

Pan, Y., Zinkhan, G. M., & Sheng, S. (2007). The Subjective Well-Being of Nations: A Role for Marketing?. *Journal Of Macromarketing, 27*(4), 360-369. doi:10.1177/0276146707307211.

Parks, M. R. (1985). Interpersonal communication and the quest for personal competence. In M. L. Knapp, & G. R. Miller (Eds.), Handbook of interpersonal communication (pp. 171-201). Beverly Hills, CA: Sage.

Patel, A. V., Bernstein, L., Deka, A., Feigelson, H., Campbell, P. T., Gapstur, S. M., and Thun, M. J. (2010). Leisure Time Spent Sitting in Relation to Total Mortality in a Prospective Cohort of US Adults. *American Journal Of Epidemiology, 172*(4), 419-429. doi:10.1093/aje/kwq155.

Pavot, W. & Diener, E. (1993). Review of the Satisfaction of Life Scale. *Psychological Assessment, 5*(2) 164-172.

Peterson, C., Park, N., & Seligman, M.E.P. (2005). Orientations to happiness and life

satisfaction: the Full life vs the empty life. Journal of Happiness Studies (6)1: pp 25-41.
Posadzki, P., & Parekh, S. (2009). Yoga and physiotherapy: A speculative review and
conceptual synthesis. *Chinese Journal of Integrative Medicine, 15*, 66-72.

Pruimboom, L. (2011). Physical inactivity is a disease synonymous for a non-permissive
brain Disorder. *Medical Hypotheses, 77* (5) 708–713.

Peerson, A. and Saunders, M (2009) Health literacy revisited: what do we mean and why
does it matter? *Health Promotion International. 24: 3 285 – 296 retrieved April 27, 2013*
http://heapro.oxfordjournals.org/content/24/3/285.abstract

Query, J., & Kreps, G. (1996). Testing a Relational Model for Health Communication
Competence among Caregivers for Individuals with Alzheimer's Disease. *Journal Of Health
Psychology*, 1(3), 335-351. doi:10.1177/135910539600100307

Query, J. L., Jr., & Wright, K. B. (2003). Assessing communication competence in an on-line
study: Towards informing subsequent interventions among older adults with cancer, their lay
caregivers, and peers. *Health Communication, 15*, 205-219.

Query, J. L., & James, A. C. (1989). The relationship between interpersonal communication
competence and social support among elderly support groups in retirement communities.
Health Communication, 1(3), 165-184.

Riediger & Freund (2004) Interference and Facilitation among Personal Goals: Differential
Associations with Subjective Well-Being and Persistent Goal Pursuit. *Personal Social Psychology
Bulletin December 2004, vol. 30 no. 12 1511-1523* doi: 10.1177/0146167204271184

Rehdanz, K., & Maddison, D. (2005). 'Climate and Happiness.' *Ecological Economics*, 52 (1),
111-125

Rejeski, W. (2008). Mindfulness: reconnecting the body and mind in geriatric medicine and
gerontology. *Gerontologist, 48*(2), 135-141.

Ryan, R. M., and Deci, E. L. (2001) On Happiness and Human Potentials: A Review of
Research on Hedonic and Eudaimonic Well-being. *Annual Review of Psychology 52*:141-166

Sarason, I.G., & Sarason, B. R. (2009). Social Support: Mapping the construct. *Journal of Social
and Personal Relationships*. Sage (26)1: 113-120. DOI:10.1177/0265407509105526

Sarason I. G., Sarason B. R., Shearin E. N., and Pierce G. R. (1987). A brief measure of
social support: Practical and theoretical implications *Journal of Social and Personal Relationships*
4(4):497–510.

Sarason, I.G., et al. (1983). Assessing social support: the Social Support Questionnaire.
Journal of Personality and Social Psychology, 44, 127-139.

Schaefer, D. J. (2001). *Dynamics of electronic public spheres: Verbing online participation.*
Unpublished dissertation, Ohio State University, Columbus, OH.

Schoormans, D., & Nyklíček, I. (2011). Mindfulness and Psychologic Well-Being: Are They
Related to Type of Meditation Technique Practiced?. *Journal Of Alternative & Complementary
Medicine, 17*(7), 629-634. doi:10.1089/acm.2010.0332

Scollon, C. N., Kim-Prieto, C., & Diener, E. (2003). 'Experience sampling: Promises and pitfalls, strengths and weaknesses.' *Journal of Happiness Studies*, 4 (1), 5-34.

Seligman, M. (2011). *Flourish: A visionary new understanding of happiness and wellbeing*. New York: Simon & Schuster.

Staudinger (Eds.), A psychology of human strengths: Fundamental questions and future directions for a positive psychology (pp. 305-317). Washington, DC: American Psychological Association.

Seligman, M. (2004). Foreword. In P. Linley & S. Joseph (Eds.), *Positive Psychology in Practice* (pp. xi-xiii). Hoboken, NJ: John Wiley and Sons.

Seltzer, M. M.; Greenberg, J. S.; Floyd, F. J.; Hong, J. (April 2004). Accommodative Coping and Well-Being of Midlife Parents of Children With Mental Health Problems or Developmental Disabilities. *American Journal of Orthopsychiatry (74) 2 pp 187-195*.

Sen, A. (1991). *The Standard of Living*. Cambridge, UK: Cambridge University Press. Sharot, T.,; Kanai, R., Marston, D., Korn, C., Rees, G., & Dolan, R. (2012). Selectively Altering Belief Formation in the Human Brain. National Academies of Science. Retrieved December 12, 2012 from http://www.pnas.org/content/early/2012/09/17/1205828109 doi: 10.1073/pnas.1205828109 PNAS September 24, 2012 201205828.

Sharot, T. (2011) The Optimism Bias: Why we're wired to look on the bright side. (E-book)

Shin, D.C. & Johnson, D.M. (1978). Avowed Happiness as an Overall Assessment of Quality of Life. *Social Indicators Research*, *5*, 475-492.

Shively, C. A., Musselman, D. L., & Willard, S. L. (2009) Stress, depression and coronary artery disease: Modeling comorbidity in female primates. *Neuroscience and Biobehavioral Reviews*, *33*, 133-144.

Sirgy, M. Joseph (2002) The Psychology of Quality of Life. Drodrecht, The Netherlands: Kluwer Academic Publishers.

Smith, B., Tang, K., & Nutbeam, D. (2006). WHO health promotion glossary: new terms. *Health Promotion International*, *21*(4), 340.

Spitzberg, B. H., & Cupach, W. R. (1989). *Handbook of Interpersonal Competence Research*. New York, NY: Springer

Soutter, A. K., O'Steen, B., & Gilmore, A. (2012). Wellbeing in the New Zealand Curriculum. *Journal Of Curriculum Studies*, *44*(1), 111-142.doi:10.1080/00220272.2011.620175

Sparling, P. B., et al. 2000. Promoting physical activity: The new imperative for public health. Health Educ. Res. 15:367-76; as cited in Phillip B Sparling. (2003). College physical education: An unrecognized agent of change in combating inactivity-related diseases. Perspectives in Biology and Medicine, 46(4), 579-87. Retrieved December 5, 2011, from Health Module. (Document ID: 475219351).

Spitzberg, B.H., & Cupach, W.R. (1984). *Interpersonal communication competence*. Beverly Hills, CA: Sage Publications.

Spitzberg, B.H., & Hecht, M.L. (1984). A component model of relational competence. *Human Communication Research, 10(4),* 575-596.

Spurgin, K. (2009) The Sense-Making Approach and the Study of Personal Information Management (Workshop) Retrieved May 1, 2013 from: http://pim.ischool.washington.edu/pim06/files/spurgin-paper.pdf

Standage, M., Duda, J. L., & Ntoumanis, N. (2003). A Model of Contextual Motivation in Physical Education: Using Constructs From Self-Determination and Achievement Goal Theories to Predict Physical Activity Intentions. Journal Of Educational Psychology, 95(1), 97-110.

Stanton, E. A. (2007). The Human Development Index: A History. Political Economy Research Institute Working Paper No. 127, University of Massachusetts Amherst, Amherst, Mass.

Stock, W.A., Okun, M.A. & Benin, M. (1986). Structure of well-being among the elderly. *Psychology and Aging, I* 91-102.

Sumner, A. (2006). Economic Well-being and Non-economic Well-being. In Mark McGillivray and Matthew Clarke, eds. *Understanding Human Well-Being.* Basingstoke, UK: Palgrave MacMillan.

Taylor, S. E.; Brown, J.D. ( ) Illusiion and well-being: A social pyshcological perspective on mental health Psychological Bulletin, Vol 103(2), Mar 1988, 193-210. doi:10.1037/0033-2909.103.2.193

Thomas, J. B., Clark, S. M., & Gioia, D. A. (1993). Strategic sensemaking and organizational performance: Linkages among scanning, interpretation, action, and outcomes. *Academy of Management Journal, 36*(2), 239–270.

Ting-Toomey, S. (1993). Communication resourcefulness: An identity-negotiation perspective. In R. Wiseman & J. Koester (Eds.), *Intercultural communication competence* (pp. 72–111). Newbury Park, CA: Sage. Troth, A.C.; Jordan, P. J.; & Lawrence, S. A. (2012). *Emotional Intelligence, Communication Competence, and Student Perceptions of Team Social Cohesion.*

UNDP (United Nations Development Programs (2012) website: http://www.undp.org/content/undp/en/home.html vanHoorn, 2007. A Short Introduction to Subjective Well-Being: Its measurement, correlates and policy uses. Retrieved from www.oecd.org/site/worldforum06/38331839.pdf *December 12, 2012.*

Veenhoven, R. (1984) *Conditions of Happiness.* Dordrecht, Netherelands..

Veenhoven, R. (1991). Is Happiness Relative? *Social Indicators Research,* 24: 1-34.

Warren, T. Y.; Barry, V.; Hooker, S.P.; Sui, X.; Church, T.S.; Blair, S.N. (2010). Sedentary Behaviors Increase Risk of Cardiovascular Disease Mortality in Men. *Medicine, Sport and Exercise (42)* 5:879-885.

Watson, D., Clark, L.A., & Tellegen, A. (1988). 'Development and Validation of Brief Measures of Positive and Negative Affect: The PANAS Scales.' *Journal of Personality and Social*

Psychology, 54 (6), 1063-1070.

Weber, K., & Glynn, M. A. (2006). Making sense with institutions: Context, thought and action in Karl Weick's theory. *Organization Studies, 27*(11), 1639.

Weick, K. E. (2003). Enacting an environment: The infrastructure of organizing. Debating organization: Point-counterpoint in organization studies. In R. Westwood & S. R. Clegg (Eds.), *Debating organization: Point-counterpoint in organization studies* (pp. 184–194). Oxford: Blackwell Publishing.

Weick, K. E. (2005). Managing the unexpected: Complexity as distributed sensemaking. *Uncertainty and Surprise In Complex Systems: Questions On Working With The Unexpected*, 51.

Weick, K. E. (2006). Faith, evidence, and action: Better guesses in an unknowable world. *Organization Studies, 27*(11), 1723–1736.
\Weick, K. E. (2007). The generative properties of richness. *The Academy of Management Journal, 50*(1), 14–19.

Weick, K. E., & Roberts, K. H. (1993). Collective mind in organizations: Heedful interrelating on flight decks. *Administrative Science Quarterly*, 357–381.

Wenger, E. (1999). *Communities of practice: Learning, meaning, and identity*. New York: Cambridge University Press.

Wenger, E. (2001). *Support communities of practice: A survey of community-oriented technologies*. San Juan, CA: Self-published report.

Wenger, E. (2005). *Communities of practice in 21st-century organizations: Guide to establishing and facilitating intentional communities of practice*. Quebec: CEFRIO.

Wenger, E., McDermott, R. A., & Snyder, W. (2002). *Cultivating communities of practice: A guide to managing knowledge*. Boston, MA: Harvard Business School Press.

Wenger, E., & Snyder, W. M. (2000). Communities of practice: The organizational frontier. *Harvard Business Review, 78*(1), 139–146.

Wenger, E., White, N., Smith, J. D., & Rowe, K. (2005). Technology for communities. In E. Wenger (Ed.), *Communities of practice in 21st-century organizations: Guide to establishing and facilitating intentional communities of practice*. Quebec: CEFRIO.

WHO (1948) World Health Organization, http://www.who.int/en/
Wiemann, J. M. (1977). Explication and test of a model of communicative competence. *Human Communication Research*, 3, 195-213.

Wiemann, J. M., & Backlund, P. (1980). Current theory and research in communication competence. *Review of Educational Research*, 50, 185–199.

Winkleby, M., Jatulis, D., Frank, E., & Fortmann, S. (1992). Socioeconomic status and health: how education, income, and occupation contribute to risk factors for cardiovascular disease. *American Journal Of Public Health, 82*(6), 816-820. doi:10.2105/AJPH.82.6.816

Wright, K. B. (2011). A communication competence approach to healthcare worker conflict, jobstress, job burnout, and job satisfaction. *Journal for Healthcare Quality, 33*, 7-14.

Wright, K. B., Banas, J. A., Bessarabova, E., & Bernard, D. R. (2010). A Communication Competence Approach to Examining Health Care Social Support, Stress, and Job Burnout. *Health Communication, 25*(4), 375-382. doi:10.1080/10410231003775206

Wright, K. B., Rosenberg, J., Egbert, N., Ploeger, N. A., Bernard, D. R., & King, S. (2013). Communication Competence, Social Support, and Depression Among College Students: A Model of Facebook and Face-to-Face Support Network Influence. *Journal Of Health Communication, 18*(1), 41-57. doi:10.1080/10810730.2012.688250

ABOUT THE AUTHOR

Dr. Suzie Carmack is an internationally-recognized thought-leader in the fields of health and well-being promotion, and mind/body medicine. Her unique approach to well-being promotion has inspired over 30,000 people from 89 countries to practice mindful movement, including the office teams of the American offices of the Pan American / World Health Organization.

As a well-being coach and consultant, Dr. Carmack has personally coached over 2,000 individuals, teams, and organizations to optimize their productivity, happiness, and creativity and she has trained coaches worldwide to use her model with others.

Dr. Carmack serves on the faculty of the Department of Health Studies at The American University; conducts research with the George Mason University Center for Health and Risk Communication; certifies Coaches and Yoga Therapists in her training programs; and inspires people worldwide to move at their desk and throughout their day through her online studio.

Dr. Carmack's translational research has been presented in over 50 keynote addresses throughout the U.S. and abroad, as well as at major academic conferences, including the American Public Health Association, the National Academies of Practice, and the National Communication Association.

As an interdisciplinary scholar, Dr. Carmack holds a PhD in health communication from George Mason University (2014); a MEd in health and kinesiology from University of Texas at Tyler (2009); a MFA in Theatre / Arts Administration from University of Alabama and the Alabama Shakespeare Festival (1991); and a BA in Communication Arts / Theatre from Allegheny College (1989). She also maintains professional credentials as a Yoga Teacher and Therapist (ERYT 200/RYT 500); Pilates Trainer (PMA-CPT), Personal Trainer (ACE-CPT) and trains instructors in these disciplines as a continuing education provider for the Yoga Alliance, the Pilates Method Alliance and the American Council on Exercise.

For more information on Dr. Carmack's training, research, workshops, and speaking engagements, please see www.drsuziecarmack.com.

Dr. Carmack lives with her fiancée Bob Shircliff and her children in Fairfax, VA.

Made in the USA
Las Vegas, NV
27 January 2022

42404833R00095